The Pink Moon Lovelies

Empowering Stories of Survival

Created By

Nicki Boscia Durlester

Published in the United States of America by Createspace

ISBN -13: 978 -1480271289, ISBN – 10: 1480271284
Manufactured in the United States of America

First edition published 2013

Created by Nicki Boscia Durlester

Edited by Nicki Boscia Durlester and Susan Long Martucci

Photos edited by Melissa Johnson Voight

Glossary of Terms and Links by Marie Flodin and Lisa Marie Guzzardi

Cover art and design © 2013 by Shera Delia

for the pink moon lovelies

TABLE OF CONTENTS

PREVIVORS

Uninformative BRCA Negative Previvor

BRCA (True) Negative

IN MEMORIAM

ACKNOWLEDGMENTS

GLOSSARY OF TERMS

LINKS

Many pink hearts of love and compassion for others create the mass and influence of Pink Moon. Of which comes a growing community of those with the courage, experience and empathy that generate a healing force and vibration for the benefit of all. Wounded Healer Archetypes organizing to make a change is powerful Sacred Activism.

~ MICHAEL PAULDINE ~

FOREWORD

Ten seconds repeatedly occur in my life. They usually happen with an ultrasound probe in my right hand, and an image on a screen to my left. The image is breast cancer, and I instantly know it. As I capture a few more pictures, I hold my breath. If I don't exhale, then she won't know what I know... if I don't exhale, then she doesn't have to start fighting for her life... but I have to exhale, and whatever I say next will jumpstart an emotional whirlwind. I already know that the tempestuous winds will calm, her tenacious spirit will rise, and she will emerge victorious. I do my best to instill confidence and hope, and for good reason - early stage breast cancers have a 99% survival rate.

I have a favorite line that patients say to me: "Well, I'm not high risk for breast cancer because no one in my family has it." Not so fast there, my friend. Did you know that only 20% of all breast cancer patients have a single relative with breast cancer? Besides being a BRCA mutation carrier, the two biggest risk factors for getting breast cancer are (1) being a woman, and (2) getting older. It turns out, breast cancer does not discriminate, and aging women represent a rather available target. Although the majority of the stories in this book are those of BRCA survivors and previvors, BRCA mutations account for only 5-10% of all breast cancer cases. For BRCA carriers, the chances of breast cancer approach 85%, and up to 54% for ovarian cancer. In my opinion, this mutation trumps all of your healthy habits and good intentions. The best strategy for carriers is intense breast and ovarian surveillance until one desires prophylactic mastectomies and/or ovary removal to maximally reduce the chances of a diagnosis. Prevention does not yet exist.

Our best defenses against cancer – BRCA carrier or not - are early detection and risk reduction. Early detection requires awareness, which, in turn, promotes vigilance. Vigilance includes annual mammograms and clinical breast exams beginning at age 40, and monthly self-breast exams starting at age 18. Despite any hogwash you may have heard to the contrary, mammograms save lives. Mortality rates (i.e., death) for women decrease between 20-35% when they obtain yearly mammograms, as compared to women who skip years between mammograms. The breast plan for BRCA carriers begins even earlier, and can also involve breast MRI, ultrasounds, and biannual exams.

Our tagline at the Pink Lotus Breast Center is "Let's Save Lives" – it's embroidered onto the front of our uniforms; it's the essence of our mission statement; it's the goal of this book; it's the purpose of my life. So, whenever I have a captive audience like you, dear reader, I feel compelled to try to save at least one person's life, and right now, that's yours. So, listen up – here come my Top 5 Risk Reducers:

1. Cut it. Alcohol increases estrogen levels, impairs immune function, and inactivates folic acid (which is important for repairing DNA when it goes awry). Keep it to one a day, lady!

2. Lose it. No question. No controversy. Obese women have over twice the breast cancer *incidence*, breast cancer *recurrence*,

and breast cancer-related *death* than non-obese women. Good news for the plus-sizes: lose that fat – *and you will lose your risk!*

3. Move it. Women who exercise for 3–4 hours per week at moderate to vigorous levels have a 30-40% lower incidence of breast cancer than sedentary women. Come on, break a sweat!

4. Eat it. Here's your healthy meal snapshot: high fiber, low fat, lean meat (chicken, fish, turkey) with an abundance of fresh fruits and vegetables (preferably organic) with a splash of mono-unsaturated oil (olive, sesame, flaxseed).

5. Forget it. Resentment, anger, depression, grudges... *Stress* creates chronic inflammation, the preferred environment for your neighborhood cancer cell. Deep breathe. Let it go. The stress is killing you.

Every time the Pink Moon Lovelies share their stories, their words carry the power to save lives. The Pink Moon Lovelies, Empowering stories of Survival represents a remarkable collaborative effort of the collective heart and soul of survivors and previvors from around the globe. Each woman found the courage to tell her story, and in so doing, she can be assured that her story will resonate with someone, somewhere, who will make a change that leads to life. One person can make a difference. My sweet, witty, unstoppable friend and patient, Nicki Durlester, has taken her message global with a singular focus: a chance to educate is a chance to cure. So, read on, and live long!

With love,
Kristi Funk, MD, FACS
Founder and Director, Pink Lotus Breast Center

INTRODUCTION

One person can make a difference. Her name was Bianchina Bus-chi Boscia. She was my muse for my first book, <u>Beyond the Pink Moon, A Memoir of Legacy, Loss and Survival</u>. My mother was an extraordinary woman filled with a generosity of spirit I have rarely seen. She passed down many gifts to me. Unknowingly she also passed down the BRCA gene mutation sealing my fate for a future diagnosis. <u>Beyond the Pink Moon</u> intimately narrates my journey during my diagnosis, treatment and recovery from breast cancer. Dedicated to my mother, it weaves our stories and priceless memories of enduring love.

After publishing <u>Beyond the Pink Moon</u> I created a Facebook page by the same name to establish an active forum for discussion for people whose lives have been touched by breast and ovarian cancer. The goal from day one was to save lives. While looking for similar groups on Facebook, to share my memoir with, I discovered the BRCA Sisterhood. Teri Smieja, the moderator, graciously allowed me to showcase my book on the group's page. I held a raffle for ten free copies to encourage the sisters to join Pink Moon and soon our membership began to grow. Also contributing to our growth was an angel from England named Wendy Watson, the founder of The National Hereditary Breast Cancer Helpline and author of

I'm Still Standing, who brought her legion of fans. Pink Moon struck a chord and quickly became a global support group for previvors and survivors of breast and ovarian cancer.

While on the BRCA Sisterhood, I was drawn to a striking young woman who stood out in the crowd because of her inspirational pink posts. When she joined Beyond the Pink Moon our members gravitated towards her. I felt led to ask her to moderate Pink Moon with me. I believe it was divine intervention. I am so fortunate that the lovely Melissa Johnson Voight said yes. Melissa is a BRCA1 previvor and I am a BRCA2 survivor. Together we cover all the bases. Her heartfelt story is included in our collection.

One of the original members of Beyond the Pink Moon, Susan Long Martucci, coined the name The Pink Moon Lovelies. She is a two-time breast cancer survivor whose brother is married to my cousin. We never met until my cousin, who I had been out of touch with for 35 years, gave Susan my book to read. She became my beacon of hope after sending me an email and sharing she was a 13-year breast cancer survivor. She had no inkling she would soon be diagnosed with breast cancer again. Pink Moon provided the encouragement, inspiration and love she needed as she dealt with her second diagnosis, treatment and recovery. Lovingly known as Martucci, Susan unexpectedly found a new family on Pink Moon and I found a new BFF. Her remarkable journey through two diagnoses is also included in this book.

From the beginning I encouraged the Lovelies to tell their stories on Pink Moon, reinforcing that every time they share their journeys they have the potential to save lives. All of their stories are compelling and have been well received on the Moon. We began saving them in our group files until one day I suggested creating a collection of Pink Moon stories with the goals of achieving far-reaching effects beyond our Facebook group and raising awareness and saving lives on a global scale. I'm not certain anyone thought it would really happen. No big publishing house behind the Lovelies. We have done it our way.

I am enormously grateful to Dr. Kristi Funk, Founder and Director of the Pink Lotus Breast Center in Beverly Hills, California for writing the Foreword of this book. I was fortunate to have been referred to Dr. Funk after my breast cancer diagnosis. She skillfully performed my bilateral mastectomy and treated me with compassion and kindness throughout my surgery and recovery. Dr. Funk is a gifted surgeon and an empathic human being who genuinely cares about her patients. I am deeply honored she contributed to this book.

In this collection of fifty stories are the riveting accounts of some of the bravest women I have ever known, who shared their hearts with courage and conviction. Included are a mother and daughter, Rosie Goldstein and Teri Smieja. Rosie, a BRCA1 survivor, has been fearlessly battling ovarian cancer for 11 years while her daughter, Teri, a BRCA1 previvor, had prophylactic surgeries to remove her breasts and ovaries to significantly reduce her risk of cancer and to avoid the same fate as her mother. You will read the gripping stories of sisters Barbie and Brenda Ritzco. Barbie is a BRCA2 breast cancer survivor, and Brenda is a BRCA2 previvor who has decided to practice active surveillance instead of having prophylactic surgeries. The most moving story for me is that of my daughter, Ally Bianchina Durlester, a BRCA2 previvor. I had hoped and prayed the BRCA2 mutation would end with me. Unfortunately it did not. It was very sobering to read my daughter's story in her own words. As a mother my greatest concern is for the welfare of my children. I take comfort in knowing

Ally has learned from my choices and will do whatever it takes to stay healthy and live a long active life.

The Pink Moon Lovelies, Empowering Stories of Survival concludes with a dedication to two of our young Lovelies who passed away during July 2012. May Smith and Linda Ritzco Cieszkowski died within a week of each other. The sadness was unbearable. Linda, 38 years old, was Barbie and Brenda Ritzco's first cousin and the beloved daughter of our fellow Lovely, John Ritzco. She courageously fought for six years against breast cancer and leukemia capturing our hearts and teaching us that in the end it is love that is triumphant. May, 32 years old, had both the BRCA1 and BRCA2 gene mutations. She bravely battled Triple Negative Breast Cancer for less than two years. Her poignant story and her final message to The Pink Moon Lovelies are included along with my heartfelt eulogy for May.

The survivors and previvors are listed in the Table of Contents in the order of their stories, concluding with an uninformative BRCA Negative and a BRCA (True) Negative. There was never a question as to which story would lead this collection. Barbie Ritzco is an 18-year career United States Marine. She discovered a lump in her breast before deploying to Afghanistan and kept silent in order to stay with her platoon. This Gunnery Sargeant put her life on the line for ours. For this reason she is lovingly known as the Warrior Queen of Pink Moon.

One person can make a difference. It all began with my mother who continues to be my muse. What began with one person on a mythical place called Pink Moon is now at over 1,200 members worldwide. Collectively we hope to make a global difference. With stories from Australia, Canada, England, Ireland, Israel, South Africa and the United States of America the goal remains the same. Saving lives!

Without further ado, it is my honor to introduce the Pink Moon Lovelies...

SURVIVORS

*People who continue to
function or prosper in spite of
opposition, hardship, or setbacks.*

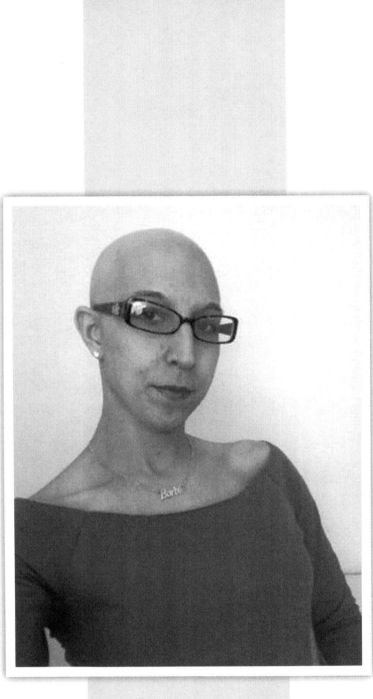

Barbie Ritzco

BRCA2 Breast Cancer Survivor, 38
Fredericksburg, Virginia USA

The Original Boobless Bald BRCA2 Barbie

by Anne Ahouse and Barbie Ritzco

Now this is a story all about how my life got twist-turned inside out,
I'd like to take a minute, just sit right there,
I'll tell you how I become the prince of a town called Bel Air...
OOPS!!! Wrong Story!!! :)

I always knew I would be the one to get breast cancer in my family. I have always been the lucky one. Winning bullshit here and there. Nothing significant but considered lucky nonetheless. I never even had boobs until I was in my late 20s, after I gave birth to my son. They were a size D. They never got any smaller; they just kind of deflated like old helium balloons. I had stretch marks all over them. I had my nipple pierced too. I have no idea why. I was in Ontario, Canada assisting with an air show and it seemed like a good idea at the time. I do spontaneous stupid things. I think I have a T-shirt or bumper sticker that says that... anyway, now all that is left of my boobs are the stretch marks. My surgeon did a skin sparing procedure. What a nice guy. Thanks doc for saving my stretch marks! He wanted to leave as much skin as he could for reconstruction since I was so skinny.

Flashback! Sorry for the flash-forward. For all that don't know my background I will just drop a few small details so this story has a chance of making sense. I am 37 years old (Italian, Polish, Russian). I am a GySgt in the US Marines. I have been serving for over 17 years. Iraq, Afghanistan, Germany, Spain, Italy, Ireland, Hawaii, Japan, Romania, etc, been there, got the shot glass. So there I was in a community shower with eight other women in the field while participating in desert operations preparing to deploy to Afghanistan. I noticed a small lump while I was washing. It was about the size of a gumball. Small in the real world. Big in the cancer world. Too busy to put any real thought into it, I just continued on with my regular day-to-day work schedule. 12 hours on and 12 hours off. One hot meal a day. Sleeping on a cot in a hut in the desert at triple digits. Eventually in a few months when things calmed down, I told my flight surgeon that I had a lump. He did what all good docs do and referred me to someone else to have it checked out. I canceled the appointment several times due to hectic work situations and sleep deprivation. We were scheduled to deploy in mid- November 2010. I once again canceled the appointment; actually I think I just forgot about it. I told my doc that the lump wasn't going anywhere. It would still be there when I got back. I wasn't going to let a lumpy boob stop me from deploying. Hell no! I went through too much to get to this point to not deploy with my Marines and my squadron.

I soon deployed to Afghanistan... me, my M16 service rifle, 50 rounds, a Kevlar, Flak jacket, gas mask, and unbeknownst to anyone else... my lump. I really didn't think much of it. There is no history of breast cancer in my family, well except for my first cousin Linda who was diagnosed at 30, if you want to call that history. I closely monitored it and when I noticed it became slightly larger after 30 days in country, I had the doc check it out. He said it felt like a cyst and he would check it again in 30 more days. Sounded good to me. A few weeks passed and it seemed to have grown again. It had taken control of my nipple. Inverted nipple... not good. I am not going to get into too many details about my deployment. I just want everyone to understand what my situation was at the time. I was in Khandahar, the world's deadliest place. I was working non-stop to support a flight schedule of FA-18 fighter jets that were constantly dropping bombs on the ground and saving grunt's lives (3/5 Darkhorse Marines). In less than 45 days, I sent 23 Marines home in boxes. Every night and several times a day, our base was under attack by rockets. We spent hours on end in bunkers waiting for a sign that all was clear. I was responsible for the lives of the ten Marines under me. We hoped all our training would work. The situation was extremely stressful. I think that is why my lump doubled in size in such a short time. Every night taking a shower I would dread washing myself because I knew that lump was there. I would cry in the shower every single time. I knew what it was.

There was no mammogram equipment at the hospital in Khandahar. It is basically a stop the bleeding point for troops before they medevac them to Landstuhl, Germany. I was told to pack a bag because I would be gone for a few days. I had no idea that I would not be returning at this point. I was briefed that if the worst-case scenario were breast cancer then they would send me home. I piled onto a C-130 medical flight headed to Germany. It took about two days to get there. We had to make several stops along the way to pick up combat wounded troops. I finally arrived in Germany at the hospital and was immediately escorted to see a general surgeon. He examined me and we assumed the worst. It looked horrible. A giant lump, an inverted nipple, and swollen lymph nodes... I was a walking pamphlet for breast cancer. He performed a core needle biopsy. The results wouldn't be available for a few days. I was lucky enough to have arrived on a holiday weekend. It was February 11, 2011. Valentine's Day would be on Monday. Great! I was able to squeeze in the mammogram and an ultrasound before everyone went home for the day. That was good news. I sat in the barracks for a few days with the rest of the wounded warriors. Some would not be returning to the combat zone. We all played the waiting game. My results came back on February 23, 2011. I already knew what it was. I was just awaiting confirmation. The chief of surgery sat down with me and told me that it was pretty much what we thought... breast cancer. I had already prepared myself for this moment while sitting alone in a room for a week. I never told anyone I had left Afghanistan. I didn't want to worry my family. Now that I knew the results, I had some phone calls to make. I guess that was the hardest part up until then. I called my mom, my husband, my sisters, Brenda and Tammy, and then my dad. I told my mom that I was flying into D.C. and they would start whatever treatment was necessary at Walter Reed in Bethesda, MD.

It has been a long year for me. I tried to remember all the details of this journey. One thing I will never forget is the hurt and pain I felt in knowing that I was not going to return to my Marine family. I trained for months with them for this. We had gone through so much. I felt ripped off that I would not be able to complete my deployment with them. I was forced to abandon them. I hoped that they would be strong. This would be the defining moment of my leadership and training. If I had trained them right, they would be successful without my physical presence. I would be useless as a leader and a complete failure if they did not succeed. In the end, they all returned home safely. Mission accomplished!

All alone, I arrived in Bethesda, MD. My mom arrived the next day. She drove down from PA. It was a Friday. On Monday, I was scheduled for the million tests and scans that we all know too well. Shuffled for weeks between radiology, cardiology, oncology, surgery, social workers, physical therapists... did I miss any -ologies or -ists? All the while, it seemed as if every person in that hospital had either seen my boobs or palpated them in some way. They just loved poking at my lymph nodes. What was that all about? With all that said, I will make this as short as I can. I was diagnosed at Stage IIIB. They could feel about three swollen lymph nodes. After my surgery, he said 11 out of 11 nodes were cancerous. Only a few of them were affected by chemo. Some hadn't responded at all. But that was the drill. My lump measured 8 cm by 9 cm when chemotherapy started on March 24, 2011. Eight cycles of fun. Bilateral mastectomy followed on August 12, 2011. I removed both not due to the BRCA, but because I did not want one real boob and one fake boob. Radiation for six weeks ended on November 22, 2011.

My next step in this was to have my ovaries removed on January 18, 2012. Reconstruction is not anywhere in my future. I have two more years until I can retire from the Marines. Right now, I can't see myself having another surgery that I consider optional and unnecessary for me. Sure boobs would be great but for whom. I have never seen things more clearly. After being stripped of everything on my body, my life has never made more sense than it does now. I felt more complete being bald and boobless than I ever had before. In my case, it isn't a matter of you don't miss it until it's gone. I do not miss my boobs and I did not miss my hair. It was more like a heavy weight or a burden that was finally removed from my body. I am free! Free of things that most women worry about their whole life! My self-esteem and confidence have only been boosted during all of this. I have never felt so liberated. I will continue to do whatever I want no matter how uncomfortable people around me feel! I will not dress up or cover up or boob up for anyone!

I have to end this now. I rambled enough. I think I have motivated myself into starting a blog or a comic strip or maybe even a short story. I mean, I am no Nicki Boscia Durlester! :) But maybe one day, if I work hard, I can be!

**In some parts of my story, I added more details than others. I guess that is just the way I see it. Most already know all the horrible things that happen during chemo, surgery and radiation. Not many know what I went through before and during my diagnosis. I just felt like that was a very important part of my life and story. Names have been changed to protect the innocent. This document is unclassified. Objects in the mirror are closer than they appear. Avoid alcoholic beverages. Apply prior to sun exposure. Wash, rinse and repeat if necessary. I was just seeing if you were still paying attention. :)

I looked at my kingdom,
I was finally there,
to sit on my throne as the prince of Bel Air.

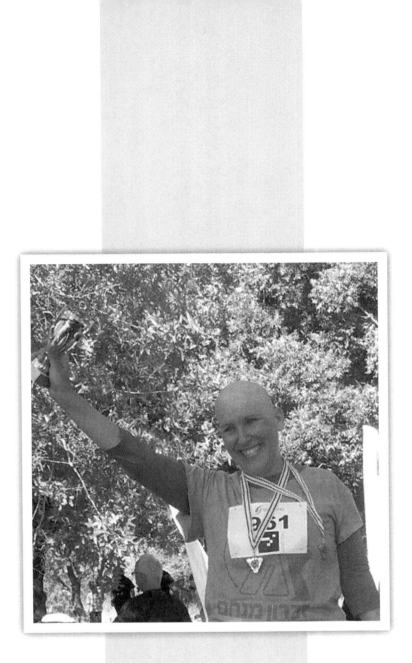

Erika Lange

**BRCA1, Stage III Ovarian Cancer Survivor, 36
ISRAEL**

Cancer Makes the Heart Grow Fonder

August 9 posting on my blog at: http://ma-ma-bla-bla.blogspot.co.il/

Here I am, back on Mama Bla Blah after months of silence. The past two weeks I feel like I've been living in an out-of-body experience. How did I get here? How does a 36-year young mother of five end up with Stage III ovarian cancer??? I can tell you it's the last thing I thought I'd be dealing with after the whole saga with the parotid tumor back in 2011. After having such a rare tumor, who would imagine that I'd sneak into another rare statistical category?

Several months ago I posted here about having blood work done and discovering anemia and drastic vitamin deficiencies. Shortly after I began to suffer from vague symptoms such as severe fatigue, morning sickness, and extreme nausea. My thyroid led us on a wild goose chase for a while due to a growth (benign), which concerned my doctors for a few months. Thank G-d; my thyroid is ticking away nicely. So why am I feeling so down? Over the next few months I returned several times to my family doctor complaining of tiredness and nausea. I felt like I was barely coping with my daily activities and life's pressures. My doctor sent me for all the routine blood tests, which were all normal. You can have perfectly healthy blood even with cancer. Good to know. Even though I was eating less, exercising, and limiting my calories, I felt like I was gaining weight! That alone was depressing and made me doubt my other symptoms. Was I becoming overwhelmed with my motherly duties? Was I lazy? Depressed?

I'll share a secret. My DH (Dear Husband) and I were hoping to conceive and each month my baby hopes were inspired and encouraged by terrible nausea, morning sickness, and fatigue, and missed periods. I will also confide that I spent a fortune on home pregnancy tests and all but one was negative. To make a long story short, our baby hopes may have saved my life! Over a period of three to four months, peaking in June, my symptoms worsened. My tummy became uncomfortable, bloated, and round. Three weeks ago, I panicked and called the women's clinic and took the next available appointment with a gynecologist on the following Sunday morning. On Sunday, July 22, 2012 I had an ultrasound and what he saw there was enough for the OB/GYN to send me directly to the emergency room. At the hospital, I was seen by an expert ultrasound doctor and referred for a CT scan. The CT confirmed disaster. Masses on both ovaries, larger than grapefruits (why are tumors always compared to fruit???) that had spread throughout my abdomen and possibly into my liver! I was hospitalized overnight.

Before being released from the hospital the next morning, I was seen by a surgeon and a doctor who told me my only option was to have exploratory surgery to see up close what the full situation was. They booked me in for surgery in two weeks time - August 8th. In the meantime, my dad did the research. He consulted with the top surgeons and physicians in oncology and found Professor Uziel Beller, a world-renowned gynecology and oncology surgeon at Shaare Zedek hospital in Israel's capital, Jerusalem. The next day, my DH and I ran to Professor Beller and pleaded that he take my case. He was on his way to surgery and said, "I'm terribly sorry that you'll have to wait two hours while I'm in surgery, but if you're willing to wait, I'll give you my full attention then..." What a relief! He went over my medical papers and arranged an operating room in two days time!!! He agreed to operate on his day off! We hired him privately. I went home for one night and came back the next night for pre-op.

On Thursday morning, July 26th, Professor Uzi Beller and his team removed all of the tumors. At first, Professor Beller wasn't able to confirm anything about the "mass" in the back of my liver. He said that he felt it and it felt soft but without seeing it, he couldn't confirm. When he came out of surgery, my family received the glum news. My poor DH and father! About 20 minutes later, the professor was able to confirm that the three liver findings were all hemangiomas - benign clusters of blood vessels. Praise G-d!

So there you have it. I have cancer. I'm 36. I was the poster girl for good health... and yet I, Erika, mother of five young children, am going to experience six months of chemotherapy and all the trimmings. I've joined a new club that NO ONE wants to be a member of - the Cancer Club, and I have to say... right now, I'm at the absolute highest peak of love and enthusiasm for life! I am overjoyed to be here. I'm scared and worried about the future and yet, I have never felt more loved, embraced, and optimistic! I'm more in love with my DH than ever before. I feel more love and joy for my family and friends, and I have discovered that cancer makes the heart grow fonder.

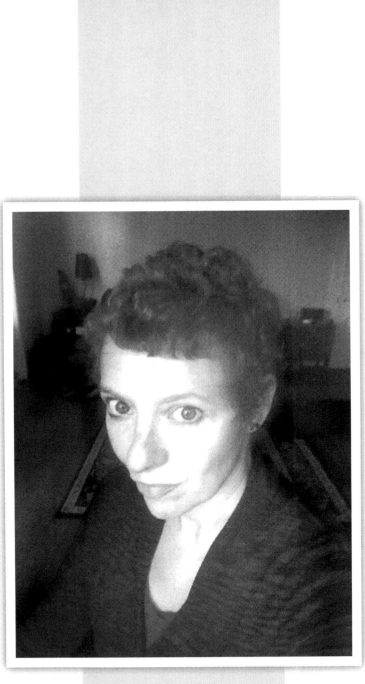

Shera Delia

Breast Cancer Survivor, 44
Ithaca, New York USA

Spring Forward

It's been one year since my diagnosis and I still shake my head in disbelief. The extent of my shock is only equaled by how common my story is. My lifestyle habits were too healthy for breast cancer. I was too young for breast cancer. I was too careful for breast cancer. With no breast cancer in my family and no friends who ever had it – it was the least of my concerns. Everything changed in November 2011. Within a few weeks, I went from a mammogram that detected nothing, to an ultrasound (given due to my insistence because of localized pain) that detected a small mass, to a biopsy that detected cancer, to an MRI that detected four tumors. With a B cup – that's a breast full of cancer. The lesson here is that I and other women with dense breast tissue could be better off with ultrasounds. Ask to see images from your mammogram – if they are solid white like mine were – it indicates a breast density that the mammogram is unable to scan thoroughly and a strong case for ultrasounds. The good news was the cancer hadn't spread and I tested negative for the BRCA gene. To quote another survivor, "I was very lucky in a bad situation."

I was also an artist in a bad situation. My artwork bounced back and forth between fear and shock and love and hope. The cover of this book, Spring Forward, is about hope and friendship -- and the special connection between women.

While I was swept away by the current of my life's events, I had three pillars of strength that got me through: my mother and father and my boyfriend who almost literally never left my side. I learned that I live in a community filled with beautiful caring friends, male and female, who shined their love on me and continually blew me away by their kindness and giving. And I learned about women, both near and far, both friends and strangers. My girlfriends kept tabs on me, fed me, brought me gifts, called, emailed, and texted me. Their words made me laugh and their kindness made me cry.

Through social networking I met hundreds of women who shared the experience of breast cancer. And somewhere along the way, I landed on the moon -- the Pink Moon. Women I've never met, from all over the world, reached out to me during the scariest time of my life. Women who knew exactly what I was going through. They knew about making decisions that their lives depended on. They knew what it was like to lose one, and often both breasts. They knew what it was like to watch their hair fall out leaving a bald stranger in the mirror. They knew about chemo speeding up the clock to menopause. They knew. And they responded to my 3 a.m. posts online with words of comfort, concern, advice, and hope. Some of these women are no longer with us. Breast cancer has taken them away.

In March 2012, feeling much relieved after surviving my first chemotherapy treatment, I invited some girlfriends over for an art gathering where I completed the painting on the cover of this book. The image was not inspired by cancer – but by all the women who helped me make it through the worst year of my life, and by my intention to spring forward in high spirits and in good health.

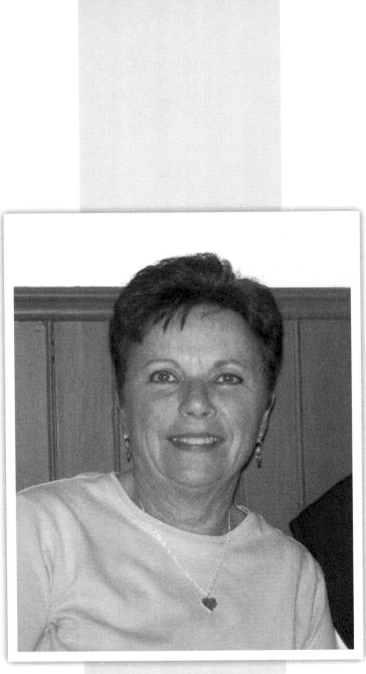

Susan Long Martucci

Two-time Breast Cancer Survivor, 64
Northampton, Pennsylvania USA

Rosebud's Daughter

It was November 11, 1997. I went to my gynecologist for my annual check-up without a care in the world. The possibility that I could get breast cancer never entered my mind – ever. I was shocked when my doctor found a lump in my right breast, which I never felt. I knew my nipple looked a little weird compared to the left one, but since I didn't know any of the signs or never knew anyone who had breast cancer I dismissed it. I chalked it up to the twenty-five pounds I lost the previous year.

On November 14th I had a mammogram and an ultrasound followed by a needle biopsy on November 28th. December 5th I was sitting in front of my new doctor – a breast surgeon – who proceeded to give me the bad news that I did indeed have breast cancer. I couldn't have a lumpectomy, according to him, because of where the tumor was located. I had to have a mastectomy. The worst news ever. I was alone, 49 years old and scared to death. December 10th I was at my next new doctor – a plastic surgeon – listening and barely hearing him describe the Tram Flap surgery I would be undergoing on December 26th. Merry Christmas Susan! I felt like I was on a runaway train and couldn't get off and desperately wanted to.

At the time my parents were 83 and 84 years old. They were my angels who led me through the darkest time of my life. The next year would prove to be the worst of my life fraught with complications following my surgery.

The day after my surgery one of my nurses gave me the wrong medication. I started sweating, my head was spinning and I was overcome with heart palpitations. I buzzed for the nurse to come and she made me wait for 20 long minutes. When she finally she came to my door – not my bedside – she asked what was wrong. I told her I needed help, something was very wrong. She sheepishly said, "I gave you the wrong medicine." Dear God – what next? I demanded to speak to the surgeon who immediately ordered a medicine to counteract what she gave me – it's any wonder I'm terrified of going to the hospital. The surgeon discharged me in three days instead of the normal five to seven because I wanted out of there so badly.

I went to my parent's home to recuperate – you know the drill... drains, meds, etc. It was horrendous. I have to insert my dog story here because it still amazes me. I had a beautiful black Standard Poodle named Spooky who was my companion for 15 years. At the time she was two and a half. Spooky loved to run down the hall and leap onto my bed whenever she could be with me. When I arrived at my parent's home that day they got me settled in their bedroom and Spooky stood out in the hall – just waiting and sniffing the air. I called for her – she walked slowly into the room and walked over to the side of the bed and licked my left hand. Somehow she knew something was seriously wrong with me and she didn't take her flying leap onto the bed that day. She gently hopped up so she could lie beside me and give me a giant hug. I miss her so much.

I stayed at my parent's for two weeks before returning to my home alone to recuperate. Those of you who have had C-sections or any type of abdominal surgery know how difficult it is to get around for quite some time. I also had a problem with my incision healing. It's a long and gruesome tale, which I won't go into here, but needless to say I suffered with an open wound until July 1998 at which time I had to have my stomach cut open again and the mesh from the Tram Flap removed. I found out I was allergic to the Prolene sutures used in my initial surgery and my whole stomach cavity was inflamed and oozing blood and pus even though I never had a fever. Just another bump in the road. I never really felt better until October 1998 – almost a year later.

I began a five-year course of Tamoxifen on February 14, 1998. I went through all the normal routine check-ups for breast cancer patients including blood work, scans, and mammograms. I was doing very well until November 10, 2010. I had two sets of pictures during my mammogram because the radiologist saw something. He suggested having another mammogram in six months and not wait another year. Okay – I can handle that. Six months flew by. On May 16, 2011 after three sets of pictures the radiologist told me he wanted to do a biopsy the next day. I was once again on the runaway train and I was freaking out. On May 17th I had the biopsy. On May 20th my doctor, in the presence of my nurse navigator, Jane Zubia, told me I had cancer in my left breast. Unbelievable! May 24th I'm sitting in front of another new doctor – a sweet, wonderful woman. Dr. Heiwon Chung gave me the news that since the tumor was so tiny (she couldn't believe the radiologist found it – thank God he did)

I could have a lumpectomy followed by seven weeks of radiation. This sounded like something I could handle much better. We went ahead and planned the surgery for June 8th. Once again I was alone and scared to death. My brother, Tom and sister-in-law, Anna stayed with me the day of the surgery and took me to their home afterwards. They cared for me until I felt I could go home and handle things on my own.

In June I met my radiation oncologist, Dr. Alyson McIntosh, who filled me in on what to expect for the months ahead. I visited the hospital many times for CT scans, mapping, tattooing (always wanted a tattoo but not the radiation dots like that!), and started the first of my 34 radiation treatments on August 1st. September 20th I met my medical oncologist, Dr. Savitri Skandan, who is another kind, caring, and intelligent woman. She explained the drug Femara that I would be taking for the next five years – an aromatase inhibitor similar to Tamoxifen but for us "older folks" who are postmenopausal!! I started taking Femara on October 1, 2011. Almost a year has gone by now. I'm scheduled for a Dexa bone scan October 10th to see how my old bones are handling the medicine.

Here I am today – September 23, 2012 finally writing my story. Yes, I'm a two-time breast cancer survivor and I'm proud to say I did it! Whatever obstacle was thrown in my way, I conquered it. Whatever went wrong along the way, I handled it. I handled everything because of my wonderful family and many friends who supported me throughout my journey. My sister-in-law, Anna, gave me the book Beyond the Pink Moon that touched me deeply. The author is her cousin and a breast cancer survivor. I felt compelled to send an email to the author, Nicki Boscia Durlester, and guess what... she responded!! Nicki invited me to join her Beyond the Pink Moon

Facebook group. Little did I know it would become a support group to me. Every morning I check on my new friends from around the world wanting to know how they are, what they've been up to while I've been sleeping. The Pink Moon Lovelies are a wonderful group of people who have brightened my life with their love, compassion and humor. What a help they would have been to me back in 1997. Because of your book Nicki, Pink Moon and the fact that we're cousins-in-law I have developed an undying love and friendship for you that will last forever and a day. Thank you from the bottom of my heart for all you have done for me. Your encouragement and uplifting spirit is immeasurable. Meeting you and your darling daughter, Ally, was a highlight in my life.

During my yearlong recovery my parents, Rose and Buddy, my brothers Tom and Bob and my sisters-in-law Anna and Frances and a few special friends cared for me. You know who you are – you're the friends who chose to stand by me and who are still beside me all these years later. You're the friends I could call on day or night. Whatever the request, you made it happen. A special thank you to my lifelong friend, Nancy Feaver. While struggling daily with her own health issues, Nan still found the time to pray for me on the phone and send me uplifting cards and notes. Her love and positive prayers meant the world to me.

Even though I was going through the darkest days of my life, God blessed me with my own special angel. She lives next door to me and her name is Mary Laky. Mary brought me meals, drove me to appointments, did my grocery shopping, shoveled my snow-filled driveway, and took care of my beloved dog Spooky. Mary sat quietly with me while I cried, put her arms around me when I needed a hug and laughed with me when we thought something was funny. Every

October Mary gives me a special breast cancer awareness gift. She never fails to acknowledge my two-time survivorship. Because of my best friend, Mary, I am still alive today. God is good. Thank you for all your love and support dear family and friends.

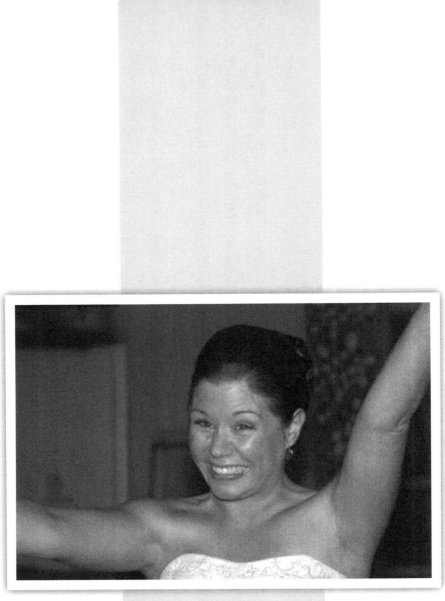

Maria Flodin

BRCA1 Breast Cancer Survivor, 32
SWEDEN

To Be Continued...

It was 2003 and I was 23 years old. I had just completed my first year as a nurse at the oncology ward and my boyfriend and I had moved into our first real apartment together. Life was busy but exciting, filled with promises and new adventures. Days flew by and I remember a not so very tidy apartment but still a fun filled little home. We used to be silly and call each other way too loud from the kitchen to the living room just to make a point of how big we thought the apartment was.

My mom lived just a few blocks from us. She had just met the love of her life and was working full time as a manager of elderly care. Everything changed on the day she found a lump in her breast. This wasn't the first time. She had a few cysts before so at least I didn't worry too much about it. Mom scheduled a doctor's appointment right away (thank God). They immediately referred her for a mammogram.

I remember that day as if it were yesterday because it was the day an ice storm threw my town into chaos. The cars got stuck in the roads, the buses stopped running and I stood with most of the dayshift personnel outside the entrance of the city hospital and wondered how on earth I was going to get home. It was a five-minute car ride from the hospital to our apartment. That day it took me two hours to walk home. I climbed in the snow on the side of the road because it was absolutely impossible to move one foot in front of the other on the ice. Rain kept pouring down which made it even more slippery. I made it down to the food store just a few hundred meters from where we lived, when I heard someone calling my name. I was walking in last summer's flower arrangements because it was the only place my feet found solid ground. For a second, I thought someone was about to correct me for that. But it was my mom calling my name. She was standing outside the food store with a black umbrella over her head, holding on to a pole. I went over to her, or maybe I slid over to her with a smile on my face (because even if everyone else thought that this slippery day was too much, I kind of liked the adventure). I said, "How did it go today?" And she blurted out, "I have cancer!" Now what happened after that I could not tell you. I know I stayed the night at mom's apartment and I know we did a crossword puzzle that night...that's about it. Now I need to try and fast-forward a bit.

Two weeks later we sat at my grandmother's with mom and her three sisters and talked about my mother's breast cancer. They also discussed their aunt on their father's side who had a bilateral mastectomy several years before due to breast cancer, but we didn't link the pieces together at that time. Suddenly one of my aunts said, "I have lumps in my breast as well, I've had them there for a while." We reassured her that it was probably nothing. What were the odds of her having breast cancer as well. Well she did have breast cancer, and that's the beginning of my story.

I told my mom we needed to look into hereditary cancer. She told her doctor and soon after my mom and aunt went to get tested. That was in 2004 and they didn't find a mutation at that time. The genetic counselor told me over the phone I had a theoretic risk of 50% to develop breast cancer and that my risk would start to increase at the age of 30. I was now pregnant with our first son. I was 24 and scared to death. I spent my days at work with women dying of breast cancer and this was a bit too much for me with my pregnancy hormones. I ended up with postpartum depression, which I think developed because of the stress. We decided to try and get pregnant because I wanted my mom to experience grandchildren. At that point I didn't think she was going to be a survivor. I also had a feeling that I should be in a hurry.

They later retested my mom's blood sample and found that she had a mutation on the BRCA1 gene. She and one of her sisters had inherited it from their dad. In June of 2010 it was my turn to get my results. For my 30th birthday (June 1) my hubby and I went for a weekend at the high coast and I remember looking at the amazing scenery and wondering what my future had in store for me. I drove by the hotel the day I received my results and I knew...I already knew...

I did have the mutation. By now I had a five-year-old and one-year-old sons. After that summer I returned to work and this time it wasn't the oncology ward; it was at Hospice. I had already worked there for a year before I had my second son. I loved it and I loved my colleagues. However I was afraid that it would be too much at this point to face people dying of cancer every day. They called me from work and asked if I was coming along on a trip to Scotland to visit a Hospice there. I was in turmoil and the thought of leaving my family was overwhelming. I stayed home and slept. I slept a lot.

I don't think I ever felt as alone as I did those first months after getting my results. I tried to have a fighting spirit, but I had no finish line. How do you run a marathon that never ends? And how do you do it alone? I had my family, but we didn't understand each other at all, and I sure don't blame them. And then came rescue!!!! Thank you Mighty God in Heaven that you always open a way for us to continue on forward...The BRCA Sisterhood! I was glued to that Facebook page 24/7. I immediately found the support I needed and made new friends (Lynda K Hrycak, I love you) and my life started to get some glow back. I was not alone in this anymore.

After that it has been ups and downs. I seemed to do alright and more then alright for long periods, just to crash when I least expect it. I went back to work and instead of it breaking me, it gave me a true sense of purpose. The mutation and the risks that follow with it have also made me see things more clearly. It is as if life is more crisp, like a cold snowy December day that pinches your cheeks and makes your breath form ice drops on your collar. However good or bad I felt there were still decisions to make. Hard decisions, or to be truthful the decisions in themselves have not been too hard. It's figuring out if I'm comfortable living with whatever consequences my choices will bring that is hard. I think I have concluded that everything just isn't going to be comfortable.

In making these decisions I found myself spiraling down. My mood got worse and I was tired all the time. I think that is one of my defense mechanisms... I just get tired. And then came rescue again. This time I found a Facebook group, Beyond the Pink Moon. I could literally write forever about how much it means to me to have a place to share and encourage each other the way we do on Beyond the Pink Moon. I just can't find all the words that description would need. And

I could namedrop like crazy, because I have met the most amazing women there, but you all know who you are!! And I love you!

In November 2011 I went to the plastic surgeon and planned my prophylactic bilateral mastectomy. He said I would have to wait, probably six months before it was my turn. Two weeks after that I did my first MRI. I didn't hear anything back from anyone after that MRI so in the end of January I started making calls to see what had happened. The results had been sent to the wrong person and when I finally got them they said I had a 5 mm tumor in my right breast that looked benign. A follow-up MRI would be scheduled. It scared me so much. At this point I could feel a lump in my breast and it seemed bigger then 5 mm. I went for my second MRI and found out I had a tumor that was 25 mm, however they thought it was a different one then the first. I'm not so sure. I was told I would be scheduled for an ultrasound, but the days came and went and I never heard a word. I called to see what had happened and they scheduled me for April 12th, which would make it more then a month from the second MRI. I broke down and cried. Luckily for me a colleague at work was disgusted with the waiting. She made some calls for me and managed to get me in for an earlier appointment. I was so grateful for that.

The ultrasound looked benign but because of my BRCA status and family history the doctor decided to do a fine needle biopsy. I didn't believe it was benign. I was really stressed out as I anxiously waited for the results. Guess what? Malignant cells!! I was very sad but wasn't surprised. They wanted to do a core biopsy, but I fought for a complete mastectomy instead. They said that wasn't really appropriate because they didn't have a full diagnosis, but they agreed because I had already scheduled a prophylactic mastectomy so the outcome would be the same. The results showed an aggressive 15 mm triple negative breast cancer tumor. The surgeon told me she had not believed it would be malignant up until she had the pathology report in her hand. Now I face more surgery and chemo.

I am blessed with the best support there is on Beyond the Pink Moon and I try to give my day over to the Lord before I get out of bed in the morning. It's not what I planned but it is my life and I will live it. I know as a human I only have a very limited perspective of things and I trust a greater plan. Moment by moment there is much to be thankful for.

To be continued...

Zelda Nagel

BRCA2 Breast Cancer Survivor, 30
SOUTH AFRICA

Never EVER Give Up

If you are looking for a story with a happy ending, don't read mine yet. Come back in about four months or maybe less. However for me it's not about happy endings. It's about a passion for peace and love and that's something that you will find right from the start.

The little c (I like referring to it like this) has always been around in my family. My grandmother passed away from breast cancer when my mom was just 15 years old. I wish I could have met her. My mom believes she won her battle and I am starting to look at it that way as well. Both of my aunts on my mom's side passed from cancer. One had breast cancer and passed away at 35, the other had ovarian cancer and passed at 38.

My mom, however, is an eight-year ovarian cancer survivor. I am so proud of the way she handled everything. My dad passed away when I was 17. My mom didn't have a husband to support her, but she never complained. She lifted me up daily, although I struggled a lot with her illness. It was especially hard being an only child.

My own journey with the little c started at 25 while I was pregnant with my little angel, Stella-Amore (Ella). I didn't feel a lump or anything, just my gut telling me something was wrong. My doctor thought I was being crazy, but it turned out that the craziness had a lot of truth to it. I was diagnosed with Triple Negative Breast Cancer. Stage III. One week after the birth of my Ella, I had a mastectomy of my left breast. No double mastectomy, because we have never heard of BRCA before.

After that, eight rounds of chemo and 35 radiation treatments followed. I lost my hubby during this time. So a new baby, new life and no husband to support me became my new reality. During that time I found out who my true friends were. I decided not to let cancer get the best of me, and every time I looked at Ella, I just knew there was a plan behind all of this. I fought for her and will fight now again.

Just before I turned 29 last December I had some devastating news at a follow-up visit with my oncologist. The little c is back in full force in my lymph nodes and liver. This has been a rough year, going through treatment with a four year old, almost five year old. She's not old enough to fully understand, but she understands enough. Some days it's hard, but I'm keeping my eye on the goal, a cancer-free life!

During 2012 a wonderful thing happened to me, during one of my hospital stays, I met an angel! She told me about BRCA testing and encouraged me to accept what was happening, but at the same time fight with love and support others wherever and whenever I can. Never have I met anyone like her. Although I won't see her in this lifetime again, she changed me. May Smith gave me the courage to keep on going.

Both my mom and myself tested positive for the BRCA2 mutation. As soon as I'm okay my mom will have her prophylactic bilateral mastectomy. For now she'll go the active surveillance route. I have to finish treatment first and then I'll decide what to do. I have three chemo treatments left and I am certain that my scan after that will be positive.

I often think about what I have learned from all of this. Sometimes your friends aren't your friends. I am so much stronger because of this. You need to keep your eye on the prize. There's always room for awareness.

I'm speaking at a ladies tea next week and will be mentioning BRCA testing. I plan on bringing this out in the open since it was not mentioned to me by any of my doctors before I asked.

I learned that we need to build bridges not walls. Sometimes it's okay not to be okay, but we must be able to pick ourselves up and carry on. We are all in this together and although I don't wish this upon my worst enemy I am thankful to have ended up here. And I will NEVER GIVE UP!*

*Sadly, as this book was going to print, Zelda Nagel, our Divine Ms. Z, passed away on January 20, 2113. She never gave up!

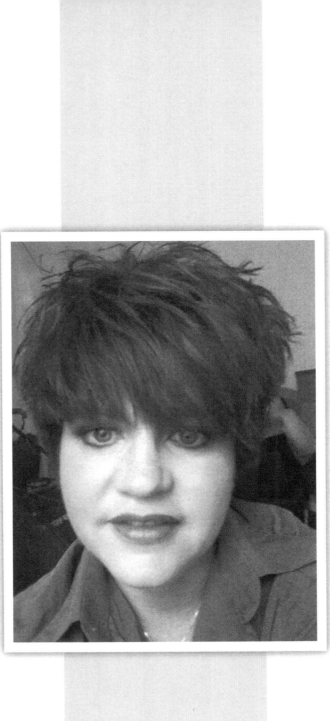

Barette Lewis

Breast Cancer Survivor, LCIS, 35
Yorktown, Virginia USA

My Prophylactic Journey at 33 years old

I am 35 years old and live in Yorktown, Virginia with my husband of almost 15 years and our son who is almost 11.

My story begins in December 2009 at the age of 32 when I found a lump in my left breast about the size of a quarter during a self-exam. I called my physician and scheduled an appointment the same day. He sent me for a mammogram and ultrasound. My first mammogram showed dense breast tissue and the ultrasound showed a cyst. I went for a second opinion and was told it was dense breast tissue and no cyst. Something did not sit right with me. I trusted my instincts and went to my physician again to discuss the results. He sent me to a surgeon who looked at my mammograms and previous ultrasounds. The surgeon did an ultrasound and confirmed the cyst, but stated it was too deep to be what I was feeling. The surgeon did not like the way it looked or felt and scheduled me for a lumpectomy two days later.

My results came back a couple days later. I had Lobular Carcinoma In Situ (LCIS). I scheduled an appointment with an oncologist to find out what would be my best course of action. I was told I had very complicated cells that were already in the 3rd stage of changing but were not cancer yet. It was considered Stage 0 breast cancer. After hearing all my options including: doing nothing except get a mammogram, ultrasound and gamma alternating every six months, take Tamoxifen as a preventative (not an option due to previous superficial blood clots from IVs) or have a bilateral mastectomy, I decided to have the surgery.

I had my bilateral mastectomy in August 2010 and my exchange from expanders to implants in December 2010. During the past year I had a couple of infections in my scar and was administered antibiotics. It would clear up but come back.

In February 2012 my plastic surgeon and I decided to do a scar revision to make sure everything inside was okay. All tissue samples sent to pathology came back with no infection present.

In June 2012 my incision opened up again. My plastic surgeon scheduled me for emergency surgery the next day to remove the implant and redo the expansion process beginning in September 2012. I will hopefully have my exchange surgery in December 2012 if all goes well.

Although I have been forced by complications to do the whole process all over again, I would not go back in time and change my original decision.

Some days are better than others, but with the wonderful support I have from my family and friends I will always push through.

Thank you for allowing me to share my story with you.

Lisa Harris

Ovarian Cancer Survivor, 49
Sparta, Tennessee USA

Appendicitis??

On July 15, 2010 my husband James made a doctor's appointment for me because I was complaining of pain in my right side. I told him it wasn't that bad. I thought I would be okay until my next day off. A couple of hours later I changed my mind and called the doctor back. He was already gone, but the Physician Assistant (PA) was there and I agreed to see her. By this time my stepdaughter came by and we all agreed it was probably my appendix.

The PA saw me immediately. After examining me she agreed it was most likely appendicitis and sent me to an emergency room in the next town. Welcome to small town, USA. Our hospital doesn't have a surgeon on staff. They were waiting for me when I arrived and took me right in. The PA came in and asked all of the routine questions. My replies were not what she was expecting. Are you having any problem urinating? No. Is there an odor to your urine? Yes. What does it smell like? Cancer. Why would you say that? I had worked with the elderly in the intensive care area of a nursing home for quite some time and that was the only explanation I could give. She kind of grinned and said that cancer was the furthest thought from her mind. She was certain it was my appendix. She ordered a Computerized Tomography (CT) scan to make sure. It's important to note that I had a CT scan in April 2010 for a severe stomach virus that was going around. At that time there was nothing abnormal on my scan including no enlargement of my ovaries, nothing.

About 30 minutes after I was taken back to my room the nurse came in and asked if I had a gynecologist. I said no. I had a partial hysterectomy in 1998 and my family doctor had taken care of all my tests. Yes, I had my pap every year. He left and said they would be with me in a few minutes. About 30 minutes later, the PA came in and once again asked me the same questions, getting the same answers. My family doctor took care of all of that and everything had been normal. She left without saying anything. At this point I turned to my husband and said, "They aren't going to find anything and send me home." The PA came back in after a brief time. She had tears in her eyes and said, "I owe you an apology. I have learned a great lesson today. I will always listen to what my patients say. You have cancer and we need to send you to another hospital now. Where do you want to go? Knoxville, Nashville or Chattanooga?" In shock I turned to James and said, "Say something." He asked me what he had just heard. I told him I had cancer and they needed to send me to another hospital right away... Tears began to flow as he looked at me and asked, "Why?" We were sweethearts years before and life had taken us away from each other. He had lost his wife in June 2008. After visiting some we were married in January 2009.

I asked if Dr. Pippin, the local gynecologist, was available and the PA explained that Dr. Pippin was the one sending me out. She explained there were cysts on both ovaries in addition to a mass in the omentum of my stomach. Dr. Michael Pippin is the best gynecologist that Cookeville, Tennessee has to offer and he wouldn't touch me. Lord what do I have?

We decided on Nashville where Dr. Laura Williams at Baptist Hospital was recommended. That was fine with us not knowing anyone personally to go to. Dr. Williams was contacted and said I could come down the next morning to her office. I was sent home with plenty of pain meds. They told me I could expect to stay for a few days at Baptist Hospital. The next day brought many tears and lots of stress. We were early getting to my appointment. I was starving so we stopped to have breakfast. I know what you're thinking, but no one told me I couldn't eat.

Upon arriving at the doctor's office the nurses were waiting and I was taken directly to admitting. WTH was happening? I was scared and didn't know what was going on. I saw Dr. Williams at about 2:00 p.m. She had seen my scans and explained what was going to happen next. Surgery followed by chemo if it was cancer. Wow slow down...surgery, cancer, chemo? Everything came to an abrupt stop when she found out I had eaten. Nice words were not exchanged and she rescheduled my appointment for Monday morning. She sent me home with strict instructions as to what I could and could not do, along with lots of pain meds.

This became the longest weekend of my life. My daughter came over and said she was going with us on Monday. My mother-in-law visited and asked what she could do and my stepdaughter stopped by and stayed for a while. Everyone was in shock. My oldest granddaughter was sitting with me on our front porch swing and asked me if I was going to die. Right then I realized that this family only knows that cancer kills. James father had died in October 2008 from lung cancer, five weeks after being diagnosed. Now here was the lady that took the place of her Nana when she had died. Was I going to leave her also? I made up my mind right then that I was not going to let this family lose anyone else to cancer. I looked her in the eyes and told her, "No, I am not going to die. I promise you that. Cancer will not take me away from you."

Surgery followed on July 19, 2010. My ports were placed on August 5th and chemo began on August 17th. I had my head shaved on August 20th. James shaved his also. That was my way of having some control over cancer. My last chemo treatment was on December 8th. I had six rounds of chemo, no radiation. I had no nausea, but was very weak. Neulasta shots made every bone in my body hurt. Having said that, I had no blood transfusions and my white blood cell count allowed me to take each treatment.

Everyone in my family went away. Only my mother-in-law came to see me. I had many friends on Facebook that cheered me on and always asked how I was. Each and every one of them learned my routine and knew when I had my CA125 done and when I would have my results. They were on the computer asking some days before the doctor called with my results. My husband never left my side. He stayed at the hospital with me, took me for my port surgery, held my hand while my head was shaved, held his breath waiting on scan results and cried with me when my doctor said there was no sign of cancer on December 27, 2010.

I go every four months to make sure that the cancer is still at bay and once a year to have a scan. So far so good. BRCA test results in March 2012 were NEGATIVE! I will always remember the day that I came to the Pink Moon. Lovelies to hold my heart should anything ever happen again.

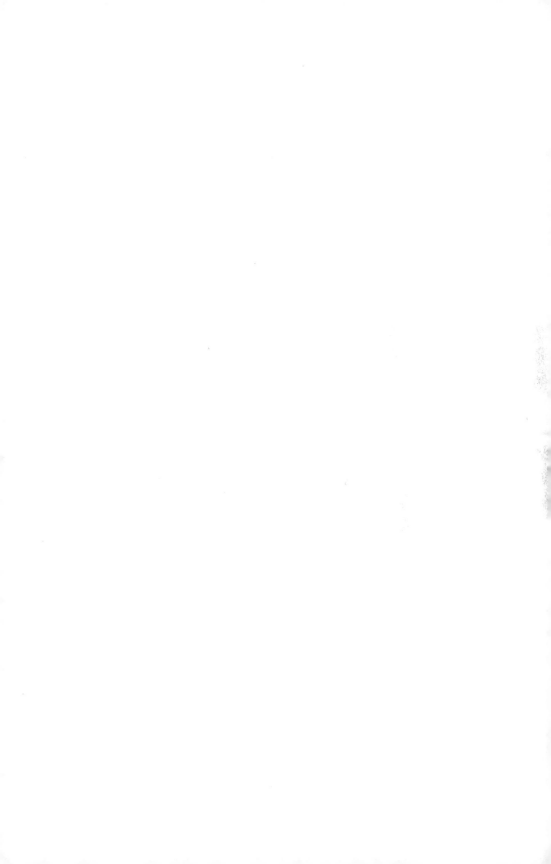

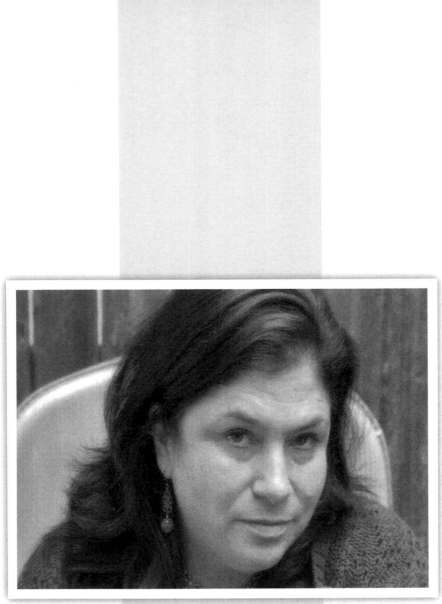

Carla J. Zambelli

BRCA Negative Breast Cancer Survivor, 48
Chester County, Pennsylvania USA

From Upside Down To Right Side Up

2011 was the year my life turned upside down. Regardless of what I am about to write, do not take that opening salvo as a pure negative, because it isn't. In fact, I have learned it is true, that in the midst of overwhelming and daunting, something amazing grows. If you let it.

It all began during a routine checkup in March 2011 with my gynecologist. I reminded Dr. Samantha Pfeifer of Penn Medicine (Hospital of The University of Pennsylvania Health System), that I had found a lump. You should understand that, for me, lumps are not very unusual. From the time I was in my late teens, I had dealt with fibroids and ovarian cysts. As my doctor felt my left breast, a look came over her face. "I'm sending you to a breast surgeon. If I miss something I would never forgive myself," she said.

I made an immediate appointment with the breast surgeon she suggested, Dr. Dahlia Sataloff of Pennsylvania Hospital in Philadelphia, PA. The day I saw Dr. Sataloff was a blur of mammograms, breast ultrasounds, and a consult that resulted in a needle biopsy.

I think in my heart of hearts I already knew what the result would be. During the late afternoon of April 28, 2011 - just as my 30th high school reunion was about to begin – I received news no woman wants to hear: "You have breast cancer." Invasive, lobular breast cancer to be precise. The room swirled for a moment. It was a total out-of-body, this-can't-be-happening moment. Then I cursed. Dropped the F-bomb in my surgeon's ear to be precise.

The first phone call I made was to my boyfriend. I just blurted out the news. I needed to know if he could handle this. He told me we would get through it together. Then one by one, I told my family and close friends. I hated making those calls.

I spent a few of those early days in front of a mirror, trying to come to terms with how I looked at that moment and how I might look after surgery, depending on the size of the mass and the margins that needed to come out around it. I also made my peace with the possibility of losing the entire breast. That was a really hard and weird place to go, but I had to do it. I stood in front of the mirror and covered up one breast. That was when it really hit me: breast cancer hits the core of femininity in every woman it touches.

I also made a major decision: I would be open and positive about my disease – but not so positive as to sound like an over-medicated Hallmark card. Already a blogger, I started a new blog (http://ihavebreastcancerblog.wordpress.com) that would chronicle this chapter in my life. My original goal was selfish: blogging would be therapeutic; writing has always been cathartic for me. But my blog soon evolved into a place for others. First it became a gathering place for my family and friends, a site they could visit for information and for reassurance that I wasn't contemplating walking off a ledge somewhere. Then, remarkably, it became a place for strangers. My blog isn't advertised, yet people from all over the country and even other countries – breast cancer patients and survivors I have never met – have become readers. It is awe-inspiring and comforting at the same time to connect with women who just get it. Because some days you just need that "yeah I know." Because they really do know.

I had my surgery on June 1st, 2011. Much of that morning was a blur but I do remember that my surgeon, Dr. Dahlia Sataloff at Pennsylvania Hospital, was in complete control and was wearing Dansko clogs I loved (patent leather leopard print) and a pearl necklace of the most perfectly matched pearls. I couldn't remember what they told me about how much of my breast had been removed, but I remembered what my surgeon was wearing and that I had had an almost exclusively female surgical team.

I had a lumpectomy – also known as a partial mastectomy – that morning. I went home later that day wrapped up like a gauze mummy. The hardest part was having to go to my local drug store to pick up my pain medication. I stood in front of four people behind the counter not waiting on people for twenty minutes before I finally asked if they noticed the woman just out of surgery standing in front of them. I think my anger was the only thing keeping me on my feet.

The initial news after surgery was good: I had clean surgical margins and no lymph node involvement. It was Stage II. A few weeks later, I received my Oncotype score, which measures the probability of recurrence. It was on the low end of the scale (the only time in my life I have been a perfect 10) so I wouldn't lose my hair to chemotherapy. I would, however, have to have radiation five times a week for seven weeks – 35 treatments in all – followed by five years on the drug, Tamoxifen.

Dr. Marisa Weiss and her team at Lankenau Hospital in Wynnewood, PA would handle my radiation treatments. Founder of the Ardmore-based non-profit, BreastCancer.org, Dr. Weiss is an energetic advocate for educating women about breast health. She gives breast cancer survivors – and women who want to be proactive about their breast health – a path to follow that is understandable, livable and empowering. She is also a survivor, which means on all those extra emotional levels she really gets it.

Radiation, although easier then chemotherapy, was still rough. Not only are you incredibly tired all the time, but you also have to live with perpetual sunburn that really, really hurts. Because my skin is sensitive, I also had to put up with what can only be described as radiation rash and patches of degraded skin. Sharp, shooting pains ran through the surgical site periodically as internal stitches continued to work their way out. Some days I was so tired that all wanted to do is sleep, but I couldn't. Still, every day of radiation brought me one step closer to the end of that phase of my treatment.

During those months from diagnosis to the end of treatment I learned a lot about myself. I learned that I'm much tougher than I thought and that I've been blessed. Not only do I have a supportive family and boyfriend, but I also have the most amazing friends in the world. Early on they decided I would never go to a radiation treatment or a doctor's appointment alone so a friend from high school, Linda Mackie, created a rotating chauffeur schedule, better known as the "Driving Miss Daisy List."

Far away friends and non-drivers were supportive in other ways. They kept me going through every single day of this. I will never be able to repay the debt I owe them.

On September 13, 2011, a sunny Tuesday morning, I finished my radiation. I was overcome with emotion all morning but did my actual crying in the treatment room when it was over – bittersweet tears of happiness, relief and gratitude. I knew I'd never forget the awesome team of technicians and nurses at Lankenau Hospital.

A slew of my Driving Miss Daisy pals and my mother, along with a dear male friend (who braved the gal gauntlet) had gathered in the waiting room that day. When it was all over and I rang the special bell signifying the end of treatment, they cheered. A hospital administrator chided us for being too loud. (I was, needless to say, unapologetic.)

My life changes did not end with the one and 6/8 left breast of it all. It has now been a year anniversary for my surgery and treatment. My life has continued to evolve. My sweet man and I are continuing our life path, together. Making a new home and life post breast cancer has extra special meaning. You know the value of the magic of ordinary days when you face something like this. I also changed my career. That was a hard decision. But I woke up one morning in February, 2012 and was brutally honest with myself that I couldn't process the stress of my job and current industry any longer, and my doctors concurred that a continually stressful career path would not be a positive situation in the long run. So I resigned.

I will admit that resigning my job to choose the path of continued health was probably the hardest thing I had ever done. But it was also the best. It gave me the indescribable feeling of having a giant weight literally lift off and float away. In the current economy in the United States this has been somewhat of a gamble, and has meant additional belt tightening, but you would be amazed at how you can indeed budget if you have to.

However, resigning and leaving an industry that no longer brought me anything but incredible amounts of stress left me open to actually trying things I wanted to do. And that is the freaky thing about breast cancer - if you remain positive it truthfully frees you from the self-imposed fetters of what you think you can do versus what you would like to try.

What I wanted to do was to further explore my photography and writing. And learn how to be a stepmother. I am doing all three, and now have a slew of professional bylines under my belt. Again, I feel once a woman has faced the impossibly hard she is indeed open to new possibilities. It's crazy, but true. Who would think breast cancer would end up in a sense being one of the best things that happened to me?

There have been occasional setbacks. Adjusting to Tamoxifen has been hard. Hot flashes, mood swings, sleep deprivation. They almost became completely unmanageable when the chain pharmacy I pick up my prescriptions from decided to change the generic Tamoxifen I was on. I learned a valuable lesson that how generics are made does matter. The main ingredients might be the same, but a difference in formulation of the binders and inert ingredients does make a difference.

Being thrown into a chemically induced menopause is not easy. And I find myself facing more self-body issues now than I did when I was first diagnosed. But I continue to push myself through the negative feelings because at the end of the day I am a survivor who can write this all down. Even if some days I wonder where all the years went and who the person in the mirror with hair threaded with gray and teeny facial wrinkles here and there is.

A couple of months ago, to close the loop on other things, I did the BRCA testing. The BRCA Analysis is a genetic test, which screens women for the cancer susceptibility genes BRCA1 and BRCA2. I tested negative for both genes and the BART test too. BART is relatively new part of the testing and looks for further DNA rearrangements that would point to additional cancers.

As I write this, it is about to turn October again. October means breast cancer awareness month and sensory overload on things pink and related to breast cancer. As a matter of fact, I really disliked last October. Breast cancer is so much more than pink rubber bracelets, t-shirts, and celebrities. It has challenged the very core of my femininity and changed my life forever.

I am just an ordinary woman. I proudly call myself a survivor and count my life blessings.

Every day that goes by is one more I get to live a healthy and happy existence. My experience has taught me to recognize other survivors and women just beginning the journey. I am alive with a terrific prognosis for a long and happy life. I am one of the lucky ones. I'm also now part of the sisterhood – women of different races, ethnicities, ages, sizes and shapes – forever bound together by this disease.

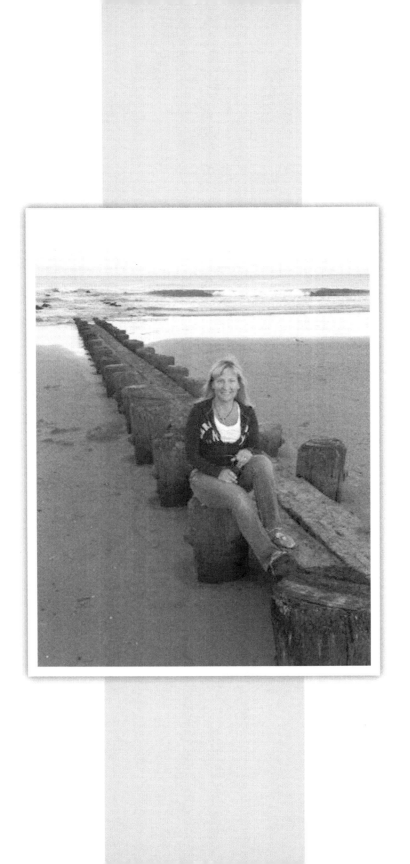

Jeanette Fanelli

Breast Cancer Survivor, 41
Vineland, New Jersey USA

My Breast Cancer Journey

My breast cancer journey began July 5, 2011, two days before my 40th Birthday. I found a lump in my left breast the previous August, but the mammogram showed nothing. After about nine months of losing weight and not feeling well I returned to my doctor. I had a repeat mammogram with an ultrasound. At that moment I knew something was wrong. The very next day the chaos began. I went from doctor to doctor and from test to test. I had several biopsies. I had the BRCA testing done and was very relieved that it was negative.

I had a malignant tumor in the left breast and precancerous cells in the right breast. I chose to have a bilateral mastectomy with DIEP Flap reconstruction. I had a 19-hour surgery on August 31, 2011. I had many complications and ended up with three emergency surgeries and seven blood transfusions.

I was officially diagnosed with Stage IIIA invasive ductal carcinoma of the left breast. The tumor was 5.2 cm, which was ER+ and HER2 -. I also had positive lymph nodes. After I was stabilized, I was able to start the next phase of my fight. I went through extensive chemotherapy. I had a hard time tolerating it and was hospitalized once. I experienced a lot of nausea and vomiting resulting in dehydration and the need for IV fluids.

I missed some treatments because my white cells were too low. After about six months, my chemo was finally over. I started radiation about three weeks later. The radiation treatments were easy compared to the chemotherapy, but I did end up with a bad burn under my arm. I started to see the end of the tunnel.

I finished radiation on June 13, 2012. After a year of surgery and treatment, I am finally back on my feet again. I was very lucky to have so much support from my family and friends. I now live on the five-year pill, Femara. It causes extreme joint pain, which affects my daily activities. I have learned to deal with it. Cancer has led me to several beautiful new friends. I would not change a thing.

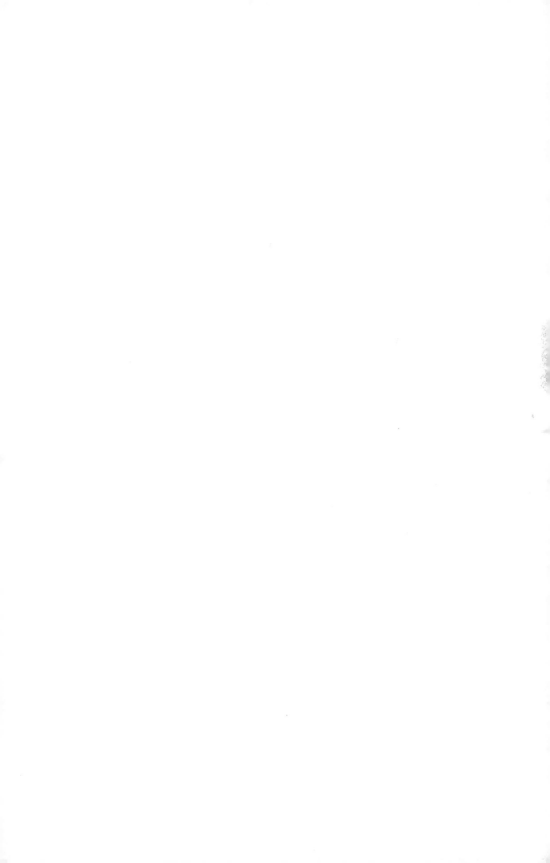

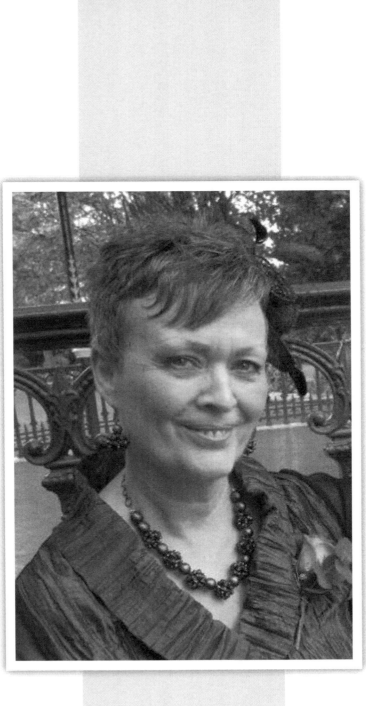

Jill Young

Invasive Ductal Breast Cancer Survivor, Stage III, 58
KilKeel County Down, NORTHERN IRELAND

The Treasures of Darkness

Cancer is not necessarily the end of your life journey, often it is simply an unexpected detour and you may be surprised at the treasures you discover along the way.

My name is Jill Young. I am divorced and live alone in Northern Ireland. I have one daughter and two grandchildren.

In 2009 I was Content with my Comfortable life; I was Confident, in Control and probably a bit Complacent. One word Changed all that, the biggest C of them all, Cancer!

No one in my family ever had cancer, at least not to my knowledge. It was never on my radar. I remember at times thinking to myself that it was one thing I never needed to worry about.

However, I was diagnosed with breast cancer on August 13, 2009. My tumor was 7cm, and 14 out of 30 lymph nodes were involved. The type of cancer was infiltrating ductal grade II, ER positive, PR Negative and HER2 Positive. The Ductal Carcinoma In Situ (DCIS) was high. I am considered a high-risk case.

I had a radical right mastectomy, and axillary clearance to level III. I had chemotherapy including three cycles of FEC followed by three cycles of Docetaxel, 35 doses of radiation to my chest and neck and 18 cycles of Herceptin; a total of 20 months of treatment. I was also put on Tamoxifen for 7 years.

Having a diagnosis of cancer immediately changes your life forever. My granddaughter was getting baptized the following Sunday and as I awoke that morning I realized I had entered a whole new world including new people, new places, a new language and new experiences.

I think the most difficult time was waiting for the surgery. I already knew that it was in my lymph nodes since one of them had been biopsied. Every day that passed I wondered if it was the day it was going to spread? Every night I prayed that God would just wrap the cancer up as if it was in Stretch & Seal and stop it from progressing any further.

I remember sitting one day, shortly after my diagnosis, looking out at the garden and wondering if I would live to see the bulbs come up. I was shocked to have cancer. I never expected to die young (well I consider 54 to be young). I talked to God about it and said it wasn't what I had expected. I loved my life and didn't want to leave it. If I was going to die I wanted Him to help me 'die well' and to be a witness for Him. I did ask, however that I could live long enough so that my granddaughter, who was only just over two months old, would have memories of me that would influence her life. That day I accepted the possibility of an early death and decided to get on with living.

In the darkness we often find treasure if we are prepared to recognize it. There is one moment I treasure which still brings tears to my eyes. The day after my surgery I showered. I still had drains in and obviously a dressing over my wound. One of the nursing auxiliaries was washing me as I sat there naked and feeling extremely vulnerable. I commented to her that I didn't know how she could do the job she did. I couldn't do it. Her words made me cry. She said, "Oh I consider it a privilege to do this for you, after all you've been through." It was as if Jesus Himself was there washing my feet.

At the time of my diagnosis I was working part-time in a Christian Community working for peace and reconciliation. I was also self-employed running an ironing service. This was a business that my daughter and I had started five years previously. When my daughter decided to leave I kept the business going, working from home and fitting it around my other job. I always enjoyed being my own boss. Working from home meant that I was able to choose when to work. If I wanted to work in my garden during the day and iron in the evening it gave me that freedom.

I have always been a problem solver and a survivor having been through many trials and tribulations during the course of my life. As far as I was concerned this was just another problem to solve. My biggest problem was how to keep my business going. I had to accept offers of help from friends, family and neighbors, which was something I was not accustomed to and found very difficult. I spoke to my bank about reducing my mortgage repayments for a period of time and looked into the possibility of claiming benefits. Unfortunately due to being mainly self-employed and owning part of my daughter's house I was excluded from any means tested benefits. I would receive some sick pay from my part-time job, but only for a set number of weeks. This meant that although I was able to take time off from my job I had to continue to work in my business throughout my treatment. I had arranged to have help with the actual ironing, but three nights a week I did a round trip of 50-80 miles collecting and delivering ironing during two of the worst winters in living memory. I was out delivering ironing in deep snow and temperatures of -14ºC. One night I had to shovel myself out of a snowdrift. At the time I had a PICC line fitted in my arm and was not even supposed to use a vacuum cleaner. Looking back on it now I am amazed at how I managed to keep going.

Ten months into my treatment I was laid off from my part-time job when the center closed. Two months after that my tenant got married and moved out. My finances took another major hit and I was not well enough to look for another job. Who was going to give a 55-year-old woman with cancer and numerous hospital appointments a job in the middle of a recession? I had a very small amount of savings left by this time, which kept me going, but I knew I had to find some other means of survival once I was feeling stronger.

When I had my last Herceptin treatment in May 2011 I cried on the way home. I was there alone, as usual, and came out and went home to an empty house. No fireworks, no one with flowers or congratulations, no one sent me a card, no one to say well done, fantastic, nothing, zilch, nada! I had been warned that this could be the most difficult time because suddenly you are on your own without all the support of the nurses and the camaraderie of the chemo ward. I decided if no one else was going to celebrate I would by having a fund raising event. To mark the occasion I organized an Open Garden over two days. My garden is listed under the Ulster Garden Scheme. I cleared out the two front rooms of my house and borrowed tables and chairs from my church so I could serve coffee. Some of my family, members of my church and neighbors came to help. The local Garden Center supplied plants for a plant stall and I had editorials put in the newspapers. Over the two days we raised just under £2,000 which I donated to Clic Sargent, (caring for children with cancer).

Once the fund raising event was over I had to turn my attention to my daughter's wedding in October 2011. I had promised to do the cake, the flowers and the stationery. This was going to take money. I went through the house pulling out all the stuff I didn't need. I sold some on e-bay and started going to car boot sales with the rest. I really enjoyed the car boot sales; I enjoyed chatting to people and many times got opportunities to talk about my cancer.

I enrolled for a half-day flower-arranging course to help prepare for the wedding. The following day I took the two arrangements to a car boot sale to see if I could sell them and recoup some of the money I had spent. I did mange to sell them but many people wanted artificial flowers, not fresh, I suppose because they would last. This put an idea into my head and I began to consider the possibility of making and selling artificial arrangements.

By the time my daughter got married in October 2011 I had done lots of research and actually used part fresh and part artificial flowers for her wedding. Once the wedding was over I began to create arrangements and went to craft fairs trying to sell them. I started a Facebook page and did a lot of networking with other crafters who are all very supportive. It was very hit and miss at the craft fairs and difficult to stay positive, but I was determined to find my niche.

The local library offered to host an exhibition of my work, which ran for about six weeks. They had a local newspaper come out to interview me. I did a free demonstration in the library and was still clearing up when my phone rang. I got my first booking for a paid workshop. Unexpectedly it was for a very small group of disabled men in a day care center. They had been at the demonstration and wanted me to come and help them make Valentine gifts for the ladies in their lives. I then began to get bookings for senior citizens groups and community groups.

I took a regular weekly stall in the market in a nearby city and the first day I was there a man stopped and looked at my work. He owned a shop just across the road from the market that sells artificial flowers. He asked me to come in and do a demonstration once a week.

I contacted organizations like the Women's Institute and Presbyterian Women and made my availability to do demonstrations known to them. I also suggested that I could speak about my own personal experience of Breast Cancer.

Right from my diagnosis I had endeavored to talk about my illness wherever and whenever I could. I realized that so many people were so dreadfully fearful of the word 'Cancer'. I had prayed that God would use me to help others. The day after my surgery one of the Breast Care Nurses stopped by my room and asked if I would go down to the breast clinic to speak to someone who had just been diagnosed. I went down with my drains in carrying my drainage bottles in a little gift bag. I sat and talked with this lady trying to reassure and encourage her.

God has answered my prayers. As I write this I am booked for approximately 35 demonstrations between September 2012 and May 2013 and at about 75% of them I will be sharing my story. I have also started a Breast Cancer Support Group on Facebook and although it is a small group of just over 30 ladies it is steadily growing. The members are from many different countries but we share one thing in common and are able to encourage and support each other.

I will never become rich in financial terms from my business, but to me that is not the only measure of success. I think it is much more important to follow your heart, do what makes you happy and live a full and fruitful life. As long as I have enough money to keep the roof over my head and put food on my table I am more than content.

BUT it was, and still is tough. I used to go to a friend once a week for tea. I remember talking about how tired I was, how fatigued and how I felt like I would never get back to normal. It is now 18 months since I finished the Herceptin and I am not back to normal. Actually I'm not sure if anyone ever gets back to the way they were, but certainly things continue to improve. Every now and again I realize that I have coped with more and feel less fatigued. Some days I feel so happy it worries me. I wonder if I am getting a bit manic, but life is good.

However, I also have my bad days and strangely my worst day came three years after diagnosis when I seemed to have a complete meltdown. This is what I posted that day in my support group: "Morning all, I'm probably going to surprise you all by having a good old moan today. I know this is probably because I am not well at the minute with a bad throat and now I have a vaginal discharge (again). But I am fed up with suffering side effects of treatment (two years on from chemo). I am sick of not sleeping because of cramps in my legs, back, neck & shoulders. I am sick of burning feet. I am fed up with my nails breaking and the skin on my fingers splitting and bleeding. I hate the sore on my nose that keeps coming back, the fact that I still have to take antihistamines to stop my nose running, the heartburn, the constipation, having hardly any eyebrows, the extra weight I now carry, the fatigue and the aches and pains in my joints. I hate the guilty feeling I get when I skip church because Sunday IS the only day of rest I get! I am tired of being broke and seeing the list of house maintenance jobs not done getting longer all the time. I am sick of only going shopping late in the evening so I can get the special offers and then eating a really weird mix of food just because it's cheap. I could scream every time someone asks me if I am all better now or have I had the all clear when I know today could be the day my cancer takes that little leap into the rest of my body. And before you all jump in with suggestions, because I know you care and want to help, I cannot afford a holiday, an alternative therapy, anything from the health shop, a special diet or anything else that costs money. So, ha ha, now you know I'm not so amazing/inspirational/awesome as you think and I am definitely not superwoman! I am just human like the rest of you and now I think I might just have a good cry."

I know that people see me as inspirational, as some sort of superwoman, because they tell me. However, I am just an ordinary woman, a woman who never expected to walk this path, but in doing so I have had an incredible journey and discovered many treasures along the way. I have met so many wonderful people. All the medical professionals I have encountered have treated me with amazing care and compassion, and I have learned so much about others and myself. It has been a life enhancing experience that I would not exchange for any amount of money.

Lisa Michal

DCIS Survivor, 42
ISRAEL

The Things I Have Learned

I would like to share with you the following words I wrote at the end of my radiation treatment in November 2011. Hadassa is the hospital in Jerusalem where I was treated.

Oncology is not a dirty word.

This country cares about its sick people and gives them so much at no cost.

There is a beautiful view from the Machon Sharet parking lot at Hadassa.

My husband is much more capable around the house than he lets on.

The children are much more capable around the house than they let on.

My husband is really there for me and in this together with me.

It's OK to go to bed with a messy kitchen.

Sometimes elves clean that messy kitchen while I'm sleeping.

It's OK to have a dirty floor, even when you have visitors.

The local supermarket does free deliveries if you spend more than 500 shekels there.

Rosh Hashana (The Jewish New Year) happens even if you haven't spent days cooking in kitchen and worrying about what you and your family are going to wear.

It's not so bad to sit in the passenger's seat.

A kind word, an email, an SMS, a phone call, a visit all mean much more than I would have ever known.

I have amazing friends that really care about me.

My family around the world really cares about me.

My husband enjoys the variety of tasting other people's cooking. Anyone want to have a meal swap once a month?

My children or some of them at least, know how to cook.

It's OK to sit down and do nothing.

When you slow down your pace you get to see things you don't normally notice.

Sometimes going out for lunch with a friend is the most important thing you need to do.

The dog is a good and caring friend.

My mother really, I mean really cares about me and loves me. (As if I had any doubts!)

There are some seriously sick people out there.

The health fund has great rights for people in situations like these.

My children really love me even when I can't provide them with all that I would like to.

The hospital does what it can to make the experience easier for you: free parking, a special close parking lot.

It helps to know a few psalms by heart.

There are more people out there than you realize that have been through similar experiences, even people you know but had no idea about.

There are amazing people who volunteer for no personal gain: helping the nurses, providing food and refreshments to the patients and their families, Hatzala, a whole big office in the hospital to help patients learn their rights that is run completely by volunteers.

It's not the end of the world if one of my children doesn't do her homework (but don't tell them I said that)

There is free wireless Internet in the surgical ward and at Machon Sharet at Hadassa.

I love my iPad!

There are so many special people who know how to practice kindness in such a way that they make you feel like you are doing them a favor.

Being with friends and having a good laugh is a wonderful way to lift your spirits.

It is possible for me to get tired of reading sometimes.

It is possible for me to get tired of fruit shakes.

They make a delicious, hot, comforting sachlav (corn flour based milky drink) at Maafe Ne'eman (the coffee shop) at Hadassa.

Hadassa is like an enormous machine with all different parts serving different purposes and it really works!

When you share with other people what you are going through you don't feel so alone.

You can become best friends with someone in five minutes when you are going through similar experiences, regardless of age and other factors.

There are some people out there who do not have the family support that I do.

There is Someone upstairs helping me, from the small things like finding a parking, to the big things like going for a mammogram when I did, going on a sabbatical year when I did and getting myself to the hospital and back in one piece on days when I didn't know if I could drive.

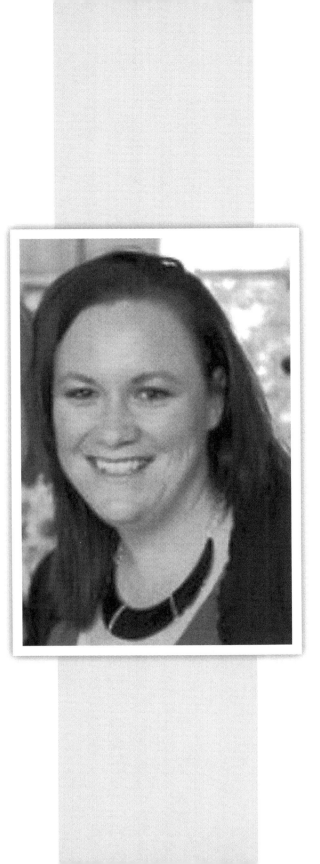

Nicole Page

BRCA2 DCIS and Stage II Breast Cancer Survivor, 28
Perth, AUSTRALIA

Lucky One

I want to share my BRCA/breast cancer journey including my challenges to have screening and being diagnosed with breast cancer after a prophylactic bilateral mastectomy (PBM).

Four of my Dad's sisters had breast cancer. When one of them was losing her battle she fought for genetic testing for our family. That is the last thing she did for us. I will be forever grateful.

Five of the seven living sisters tested positive for BRCA2, as did my dad. My two older cousins tested negative and then came my turn. I was 23 (2002) when I received my BRCA2 positive result. My doctors said there was no way I was at risk until 35, 33 at the absolute earliest! Being young and naive I believed them and continued on with my life as usual, with the plan to have a PBM with reconstruction some time after my 33rd birthday. In the meantime I would have yearly mammograms.

When I was 25 I traveled to London on a two-year working visa, with letters in my suitcase from the familial cancer team recommending an annual mammogram. The first year the doctors at a hospital in London told me I didn't need it. They said I was too young... blah, blah, blah. I convinced them otherwise and had the test. They said they were only doing it for baseline data. Twelve months later we had the same argument, however I did not win this time. They would not do a mammogram. I was not too concerned as I was returning to Australia three months later. I rang ahead and booked a mammogram on my return.

As that date grew closer my appointment was postponed for another six weeks. As the new date grew closer my appointment was again rescheduled with the excuse that there was not enough staff to run the at-risk familial cancer clinic. (Ummm HELLO – at-risk-should be a priority!)

In April 2007 nine months after it was due and three weeks before my 28th birthday, I finally went in for my mammogram. Unbelievably I again faced that same argument. You are too young. You do not need the test...blah, blah, blah!!! I refused to leave the hospital until I had the test. Reluctantly the radiographer did her job. Everything seemed perfectly normal as I waited for the results to be checked by a doctor. When two doctors walked into the room with some old scans from years before I knew something was wrong. They had found a change.

That afternoon after trying on wedding dresses all morning (having met the man of my dreams in London and convincing him to move to Australia and marry me), I had a biopsy taken of my right breast. The following day I was told that I had Ductal Carcinoma In Situ (DCIS), Stage 0 breast cancer. The recommendation I was given was to have a lumpectomy. I chose bilateral mastectomy and reconstruction. I had my surgery in May 2007, two days after my 28th birthday. Recovery for me went smoothly and I was back at my job teaching after six weeks. When I went back to my surgeon for my pathology results he told me that the type of cancer I had was extremely aggressive. Had I not had that mammogram when I did things would have been very different for me. Thankfully I had private health insurance and had the surgery within weeks of finding the lump. Had I been on a waiting list for the surgery the outcome would have been more drastic.

In January 2008 my husband and I married. In May 2009 we had our first child. I had been given the all clear and was told there was no way I was at risk of ever having breast cancer again. All was well and happy in our world until one day when my son was four and half months old. I found a lump in that same right breast while in the shower. It took me two days to believe it was real and then I went straight to my general practitioner who ordered an ultrasound. I went back to him the following day and was told it was a cyst, but further investigation with fine needle aspiration was recommended given my history. He sent me straight to my breast surgeon. The look on my surgeon's face when he read the report and felt the lump for himself was shattering. He opted not to do the fine needle test for fear of piercing my implant and instead sent me into surgery to remove the lump. He wanted it out – whatever it was.

Within two weeks I was given the news that it was not a cyst. It was Stage II breast cancer. I had a number of tests and scans to rule out secondary cancers. I also had more surgery to make sure he had removed everything. I began chemotherapy followed by radiotherapy and Tamoxifen. I was devastated at the thought of losing my hair, and on reflection I realize I was more at ease with losing my breasts than my hair!

Twelve months after I had my last chemo I was given permission to stop Tamoxifen to try to have another baby. I am happy to report my miracle baby girl was born in January 2012. After she was born I had surgery to my right breast to repair damage that was done to my reconstructed breast during radiotherapy. It will never look as nice as my left breast, but it bears my scars and is a part of my story. My husband and family and friends have been an amazing support to me. I could not have gotten through it all without them.

I taking Tamoxifen again and will continue for at least another four years. I had my fallopian tubes removed at the end of August 2012 to reduce my risk of ovarian cancer. My specialist recommends removing my ovaries and uterus by the time I am 45. I told him I would be back before I'm 40 ... I'm not letting the odds beat me again!!

Believe it or not the whole drama of having cancer and chemo with a six-month-old baby is so far behind me. It feels like a very distant memory. I do not live in constant fear of it happening again. However I don't think I will ever believe that it won't happen again. I have been told that once before. I hope and pray every day that my two beautiful children will test negative to the BRCA gene mutation and will never have to go through anything like this.

Whenever people hear my story and find out I had breast cancer after a bilateral mastectomy – they always say that it is not possible. How did that happen? It is a rarity. I guess I'm one of the 'lucky ones'.

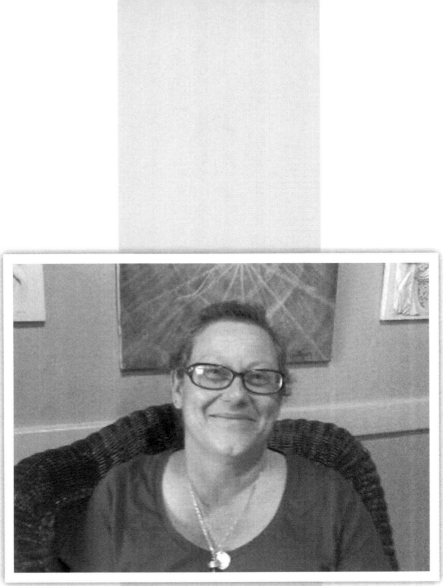

Marlene Kuma Gutierrez

BRCA1 Survivor/Previvor, 52
Guadalupe, California USA

My Introduction to the BRCA Gene

I was adopted when I was a little over a month old so I never knew my biological family. I still don't. In the last year I have learned a lot about the BRCA gene, breast cancer, and passing something on to my children that I wasn't aware of until now.

I knew I didn't fit in with the family who adopted me. My five siblings were all towheads while I had very dark hair. Mom and Dad couldn't have kids of their own (or so they were told) so they adopted me and my sister, Eileen. They were in the process of adopting another child when lo and behold Mom found out she was pregnant. My siblings Mary Anne, John, Tim and Becky are living proof of miracles. Life was pretty good for us. I was blessed to have such a wonderful and large adopted family.

I was a rebellious teenager and at age 16 gave birth to a beautiful baby girl. Joanne may have been born "out of wedlock" but not out of love. Being adopted I decided I would raise her myself. Her father and I were married a little over a month after she was born. Unsure of how to raise a baby and how to be a wife while trying to keep up with high school was too much for me. I dropped out of school. Things happened and we quickly divorced.

My second marriage was to a sailor who fathered my wonderful daughter, Michelle, and handsome son, Jeffrey. Before I could legally drink I had married twice and given birth to three children. We moved away from my family and roots in Pennsylvania to California where I found myself in an abusive marriage. I tried to make a go of it for 14 years. I was beaten down emotionally, but still found the strength to finally leave. I did not, however, address the issues of abuse and soon repeated the same mistakes. I allowed myself to be a victim again and used drugs and alcohol as a way to cope.

Years later while in legal trouble and beaten down once again, a kind police officer asked me if I wanted to go to a women's shelter. I could see the two paths before me and choose to go. I learned about the cycle of violence and how to take care of myself. I had become hooked on drugs and alcohol as a way to bury my feelings. This habit continued for several years until I reached the breaking point and sought a way out. I discovered my spiritual path. I am so grateful I found my way prior to my cancer diagnosis. I believe I would have drowned my cancer fears in alcohol and may not have come out of the bottle again. I began in earnest to recover from my addiction and have been actively involved in recovery for 11 years as of July 2012. I met my loving supportive husband of three years in recovery.

Life was finally back on autopilot when I received one of those calls you least expect, but is always in the back of your mind. It was November 2011. I was told to come in for another mammogram. They noticed a change from the previous year. Heart pounding and anxiety ridden, I asked a girlfriend to come with me to the next appointment.

Yes, there was something there. The ultrasound showed it also. I had to schedule a biopsy. I knew it was serious. My doctor felt nothing during my annual exam nor had I felt anything. Fortunately, I was able to schedule the biopsy within a couple of days. My husband went with me.

At 5 minutes before 5 PM on December 14, 2011 while sitting at work, I received that phone call – the one you never want to get. It was my doctor on the other end. "You have breast cancer." This cannot be happening. I had tickets to fly back home to spend Christmas with my whole family for the first time in over 30 years. How can I get on a plane knowing I have cancer? Am I going to die? What do I do?

My doctor's office called in some favors and got me in the next day to see the breast surgeon. The plan was to do a lumpectomy followed by radiation. She had a slot open on December 23. It was so difficult calling my parents to tell them I wasn't coming home for Christmas because I had cancer. We had lost my sister Eileen many years before. I didn't want to worry them. I remember thinking I will go home in a few months after I'm healed. Surgery went well and I had clear margins. I was home recuperating when the phone rang on the evening of the December 29th. It was my sister, Mary Anne. My dad had suddenly passed away. The next day I was on a plane back home. I am angry that cancer robbed me of my last chance to spend time with my father. But I know my Dad would have wanted me to take care of myself. I miss him very much.

Upon returning from the funeral I had the Oncotype DX test. I was informed I had a high risk for the cancer returning. Chemotherapy followed by radiation was now the revised course of treatment. Chemotherapy frightened me. I had heard too many bad things about it. I had watched my dear friend, Lynda, go through chemo for her lung cancer until she succumbed to the disease.

At some point during my journey I remember my breast surgeon telling me about a test to determine if I had hereditary breast cancer. I agreed to do it, but didn't think much about it. I didn't realize the far-reaching effects this simple blood test would have. After battling insurance to get it approved, I found out that I tested positive for the BRCA1 mutation. I was devastated to find out my cancer was hereditary. For so many years I wondered where our blue eyes came from and other genetic traits and now to receive this news. My breast surgeon's recommendations were a bilateral mastectomy and oophorectomy. I finished chemo and had my breasts and my ovaries removed.

My surgeon also suggested that my children be tested for the BRCA1 mutation. I am proud that both of my daughters had very little hesitation to be tested. My son, however, is not ready to face this hurdle. Unfortunately, both of my daughters tested positive for the BRCA1 mutation. I am just so thankful they did not hesitate to have an oophorectomy to reduce their risk of ovarian cancer. I worry about my nine biological grandchildren and whether or not the mutation has been passed down to them. I am very open and honest with them.

Along my journey I met some absolutely phenomenal women on the Facebook group, Beyond the Pink Moon, who have helped me more than I can say to walk through this. I never knew this mutation existed but now that I do, I know that I am blessed beyond words to have so many walk with me. In recovery I learned that it is one day at a time. It is not just a cliché to me. It is how I live my life.

I don't know what the obstacle I climb over today will become tomorrow. A phrase that keeps me going is "the seemingly bad versus the seemingly good". Only my God knows what He has in store. I have transformed from a victim of domestic violence to a peer counselor and volunteer at the shelter where I once lived. I reach out and support other women working on overcoming their addictions. I know that my breast cancer diagnosis and BRCA knowledge will be put to good use.

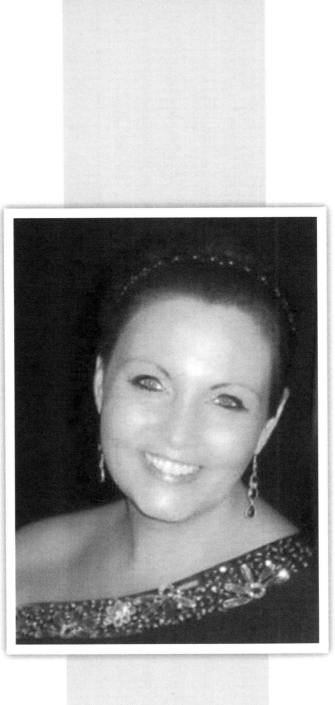

Tracey Pimlott-Grogan

Breast Cancer Survivor/Thriver, 32
Dublin, IRELAND

My Body Betrayed Me

I am coming up on my 32nd birthday. I'm a mother of two and married nearly nine years now. I live in Dublin, Ireland.

On March 2, 2010 at the age of 29 I was diagnosed with Stage IIB breast cancer, Grade III, 7cm, ER+, one node positive. Given I had no family history I was never tested for the BRCA genetic mutation. I had two operations including a lumpectomy of the left breast that did not yield clear margins, followed by a single mastectomy. I also underwent chemotherapy, radiation and drug therapies. On August 29, 2011 I had a DIEP flap reconstruction. The surgeon also removed more tissue, and I finally received the all clear. NED, no evidence of disease at last!

I will be checked regularly for recurrence. Cancer will always be part of my life, but for now, God willing, I am cancer free for good. Through this journey I have learned that I have an amazing husband, family and friends. I am stronger than I thought and I have found a voice that I didn't know I had. Don't sweat the little things. Enjoy life to the fullest.

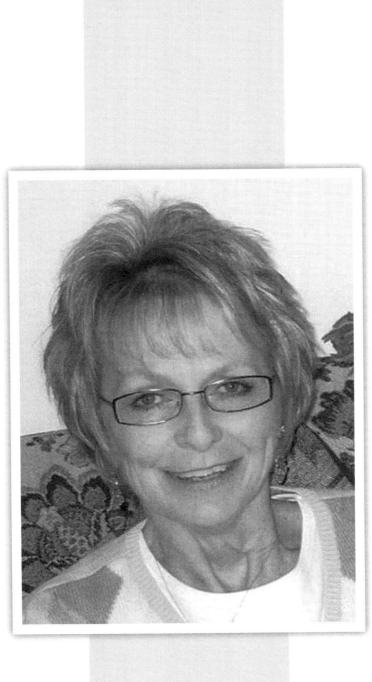

Debby Lupo Livingston

Breast Cancer Survivor, 57
Newport News, Virginia USA

My Story of Breast Cancer

September 11, 2003 I had my yearly mammogram. Results showed nothing suspicious, just dense tissue. That was good news! About a month later I began having some problems with my left nipple – a little discharge and crustiness. I really didn't think anything bad about it.

Shortly after during my yearly physical, my doctor advised me to try some cortisone cream or ointment on it and let her know if it helped or not. I used the ointment for about two to three weeks without improvement. I made an appointment to return to my doctor who, in turn, immediately sent me to a surgeon to get it checked out. If it proved to be nothing, then I would be sent to a dermatologist.

My appointment with the surgeon was on December 15, 2003. She was a very nice, down-to-earth doctor. She checked out the area and found a lump just behind the nipple. She scheduled me for a biopsy. She felt the nipple problem and lump were related. My appointment for the biopsy was scheduled at Mary Immaculate Hospital on

December 22. The lump was large and the doctor decided to remove the whole thing instead of just taking a biopsy. I had to have general anesthesia. Everything went well, even though it takes me a while to wake up after being put under.

On Sunday, December 21, the night before the procedure was to be done, I could not sleep. After tossing and turning I chose to get up and talk to the Lord. I told Him my heart's desire about the situation, but I didn't make any promises that later I might fail to keep. I did ask Him to let me be a testimony to others no matter the outcome. I had already told my husband, Gary, that I was not afraid and had such a peace about the whole situation even if it was bad news. I would just accept it and do whatever was needed to get better. He thought that was a great attitude to have. I'm also sure my attitude helped him to cope better.

I had always had a fear of getting breast cancer because my older sister, Libby, had it years before. She did not survive. She died at 46 – two weeks before her birthday. The Lord had given me such a great sense of peace in my heart. I didn't have the fear I thought I might have or the uneasiness of not knowing what the results would reveal. Philippians 4:6-7 (NAS) says, "Be anxious for nothing, but in everything by prayer and supplication with thanksgiving let your requests be made known to God. (7) And the peace of God, which surpasses all comprehension, will guard your hearts and your minds in Christ Jesus."

On December 23 I returned to work. It was also Gary's 52nd birthday. I had found out that one of my co-workers had gone through breast cancer four years earlier including mastectomy, chemo and reconstructive surgery. She was a big encouragement for me. When I got home from work that afternoon and checked the caller ID, I saw the doctor's office had called. I asked Gary what they had said. He said it was cancer and I needed to call my doctor to set up a consultation. I must say when I received that news I did get a sinking feeling within my heart. I didn't cry and never did throughout my whole journey. After calling the doctor, I began calling my family and closest friends to tell them of the news and request prayer.

What a bummer of a birthday present for my husband! That night we still celebrated his birthday and he opened his presents. Our family had already planned on going to Coleman's Nursery that night since that would be their final year. They would be closing their doors after 30 years of bringing joy and happiness to children of all ages. We had been taking our three children there since they were little. They loved seeing all the Christmas decorations, Christmas village scenes, larger than life stuffed animals, the smell of real Christmas trees, hot apple cider and of course seeing Santa! They also loved the candy store. Coleman's Nursery is a memory they will never forget.

I waited until after Christmas to send an email to my church family. Once I sent it, I received so many encouraging responses offering prayer and support during the months ahead. It is wonderful to belong to a loving church family as well as my own loving immediate family. We had a great Christmas despite the bad news I had received and also the absence of my sweet Mama. She had passed away in August 2003. I am thankful for God's perfect timing in all things. My mother was elderly and in failing health. It would have been very difficult for her to see me going through cancer and not be able to help me physically. She would have definitely bathed me in prayer. She was such a godly woman and had a strong faith in the Lord. She showed it time and time again through the years of sickness and the loss of many loved ones including her husband, son, daughter, and grandson. I never saw her become bitter or angry with the Lord. She became stronger because of it. I thank God for her and her testimony.

Speaking of God's perfect timing, on December 28, our pastor preached the last sermon on the names given to the Lord. He had preached on Isaiah 9:6 three weeks earlier but time-wise was unable to finish. The last name given was "Prince of Peace." It was perfect for us to hear that. I had already experienced peace that week even in the midst of what should have been turmoil. It is great to have a God that loves me and would be with me through my journey with cancer. Gary and I thanked our pastor for his sermon. He had called earlier in the week to tell us that he and his wife would be praying for us.

At my consultation visit with my surgeon, she did give us some good news! She said the cancer (which was called Paget's disease) had been found in the earliest stages and that it was completely curable! We were very happy to hear that. Family members were also happy to hear that as well. I certainly wanted to be a testimony and an example to my children so that when they face bad circumstances in their lives, they would have complete faith and trust in the Lord.

My surgery was scheduled for January 22, 2004. My appointment with my plastic surgeon went very well. He would do immediate reconstruction right after my mastectomy. A few days before my surgery, my sister, Vivian, found out that the lump she had biopsied was also cancer. Hers was ductal carcinoma. We were shocked that we both had cancer at the same time. I assured her we would go through this together with the Lord's help. She used the same doctors as I did. Since my two sisters and I all had breast cancer, the doctor suggested that I be tested for the breast cancer gene mutation. Thankfully I was approved by my insurance company since this test is costly. I was BRCA negative. Even though it came back negative, my children will have a higher percentage of getting breast cancer just because of our family history. But that's totally in the Lord's hands, not under my control.

On January 20, 2004 I went to see my oncologist to discuss my chemotherapy treatments. I would be getting Adriamycin/Cytoxan (AC) and also a few treatments of Taxol. I ordered my wig for when my hair would eventually fall out.

My mastectomy was done on Thursday, January 22. I felt pretty rough afterwards. I kind of felt like I had been hit by a Mack truck! I slept all day finally waking around 7:45 p.m. and was able to get up and go to the bathroom. Poor Gary slept in a chair beside my bed. I'm sure he didn't sleep much though. By Friday, I felt much better. I ate breakfast, washed up and brushed my teeth, and put on my makeup. I looked much better, too. The doctors came by around noon and both said I looked like I could go home that day if I felt like it. I went home around 7:00 p.m. that evening. Also, the surgeon told me that even though earlier she had removed the lump during the biopsy, it had grown back and was larger than before!

My sister's surgery was scheduled for Friday, January 30, 2004. She had a lumpectomy followed by chemo and radiation. I went to be with her on the day of her surgery. She did very well. After her surgery she stayed at our house for a couple of days. My church, as well as friends and co-workers, brought in meals for us. This was such a blessing. I went back to work one week after my surgery. She did very well through her chemo treatments and radiation. I give God all the glory for answering prayers and for His faithfulness!

Before my chemo treatments started I had a port placed just under the skin in my chest, which is wonderful. It protects your veins from having to be punctured each time you receive a treatment. On Thursday, February 5, I had my first chemo treatment. Everything went well. I was given Benadryl to offset any allergic reaction I may have. Thankfully, I did not have any. I slept through my treatment because the Benadryl made me so sleepy. Gary was with me. It took several hours. Before going for my treatment I took my medication for nausea, which was suggested by the doctor. I did really well, but by Saturday I was really tired and had to continue my nausea medication. I had my treatments every other week and they were always on a Thursday. I was able to go back to work on the following Monday. After my second treatment, I noticed my scalp had a tingling sensation. Then daily my hair began to fall out. Little by little, it was on my bed pillow and everywhere so I cut it really short. About a week later I went to a beauty salon and the hairdresser shaved my head. They did that free for breast cancer patients. It never really bothered me that I lost my hair because I knew it would grow back.

After three or four treatments, I requested not to be given the Benadryl. I did fine without it and was actually able to drive myself to and from the oncology office where I received my treatments. I went by myself so Gary did not have to miss work. He was so good to me and would have done anything to help me. I am so glad to have had his love and support and that he was there for me during that time.

I finally finished all my treatments! Didn't miss any scheduled ones due to low blood counts! Praise the Lord!! About a year later, my oncologist heard about a new cancer preventative medication called Herceptin. My type of cancer was HER2 positive (Human Epidermal growth factor Receptor) which meant that my cancer was aggressive, but it was not estrogen and progesterone hormone positive. My sister's was hormone positive so she was a good candidate for

Tamoxifen. That would not help me and Herceptin would not help her since our cancers were different. I was given a weekly Herceptin IV for one year. Did very well with that and had no side effects at all. Herceptin can affect the heart; so periodically throughout the year I had to have a MUGA scan that checks how strong the "squeeze" of your heartbeat is. Thankfully mine was always good.

My sister and I have been CANCER FREE since then!! I pray that I stay cancer free, but it's not something I fret over or worry about. My faith and trust is in the Lord Jesus Christ. If He chooses to allow cancer to return, I know that He will be with me again just as He was before. I never cried over having cancer. Tears of joy came only when I thought of how faithful God was to me during my journey with breast cancer.

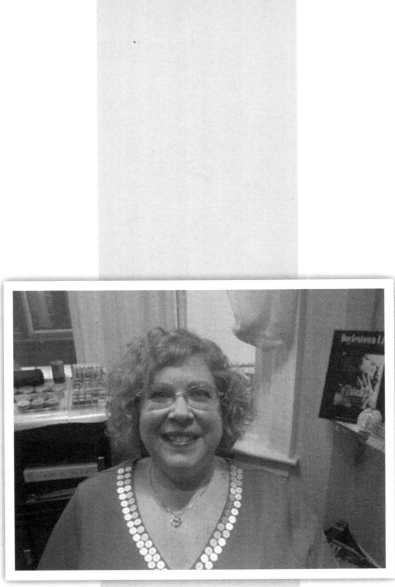

Beth Weiner Pfeiffer

BRCA2 Survivor/Previvor, 53
Willow Grove, Pennsylvania USA

Thankful For My Genes

To start, here is a poem I wrote that was included in the FORCE 10th Anniversary book:

I am thankful for my genes.

They make me what I am today.

I am cancer-free because I chose to know.

I am cancer-free because I chose to lose the parts that would give me trouble.

I am cancer-free because I chose life over death.

I am cancer-free because my genes don't control my life.

My debacle with the BRCA2 genetic mutation began as far back as my paternal great-grandmother. As far as we know she had breast cancer. My grandmother whom I am named for had breast cancer in the mid-1940s. My father was diagnosed with breast cancer in 1984 and passed away in 1989. It is from my father I inherited my genetic mutation. All of my grandmother's sisters had bouts with breast cancer. Only their baby sister had been diagnosed as a young woman.

Additionally two of my dad's cousins had ovarian cancer. Yes, ladies and gentlemen, my father's side.

Perhaps in today's medical climate my father's bout with thyroid cancer in the 1960s may have thrown up a red flag. Today we would have been tested due to our staggering history of cancer in addition to being from an Eastern European Ashkenazi Jewish background. But I am getting ahead of myself.

I began in my twenties to get mammograms way before it was standard of care for someone with the BRCA mutation. Of course the paperwork at the breast center never had a place to check off 'father' as the breast cancer side. It was not something even considered. Each one of the technicians and nurses told me not to worry if it was from his side of the family. I was already trying to educate people without even knowing at the time there was a demon lurking in my makeup. The genetic mutation had not been identified.

Fast-forward a bit. My father went through chemotherapy every week to treat his breast cancer followed by Tamoxifen to prevent metastatic disease. Fortunately we had a family furniture business at the time. If he needed to he could slow down or take a nap in a chair. His veins became calcified very quickly so they installed a port, something that is standard of care today. The cancer eventually progressed into his bones. The doctors tried a "Hail Mary" play and removed his testicles to stop the estrogen production as much as possible.

I am amazed to this day how my father suffered through the pain, sickness and humiliation of his treatments. He was always so stoic and never complained. If he did it was never in front of my younger brother or me. With the treatments that were available at the time, our dad made it to their 30th wedding anniversary and my brother's graduation in the top 10 of his class from William Penn Charter School in 1987. He also slowed down and appreciated his time with us and took vacations, which he never did before. When my parents took my brother to Amherst College, my dad helped unpack as much as my mom and my brother would let him. Then he and my mom spent a week at a bed and breakfast in Connecticut to share some time alone.

My father missed so much after his death in 1989 including my brother's college and law school graduations, my brother's wedding and mine, the births of his three grandchildren, my son's Bar Mitzvah and high school graduation. I think of all the gatherings he is missing. Because we worked together we were even closer than most fathers and daughters. He and I had a special relationship. It was his wisdom and advice I always sought first. I am grateful he was with us for so long. The doctors had given him six months and through their efforts he was here another four years.

Fast forward to 1996. My uncle, dad's brother, got us involved in a study at Fox Chase Cancer Center (FCCC). This was the first of its kind. I did not fully comprehend what it all entailed but after five vials of blood and several weeks of waiting, we got the results. All who tested, including my dad's frozen pathology sample, came back BRCA2 positive. I spent several sessions talking and crying with the genetic counselor at FCCC. We mapped out a plan. For now I would practice strict surveillance. That entailed twice yearly breast checks, once with a gynecologist and once with a breast specialist, yearly CA125 blood test for ovarian cancer and a yearly Transvaginal Ultrasound (TVUS). Ugh, I hated the TVUS. Humiliating at best, uncomfortable at worst with having to drink and hold so much liquid. Funny note, the breast specialist is a noted doctor I had a crush on in 10th grade. At our first visit I was so embarrassed when I realized I was being felt up by my teenage crush.

In 2002 after a divorce and meeting my husband-to-be, my breast specialist suggested removing my ovaries prophylactically or as he put it, "Get rid of the ticking time bombs." At 42 I did not want more children and had an "AHA" moment when babysitting my six-month-old niece. I was not doing the baby thing again. I opted for bilateral removal of my ovaries. A snap operation! Laparoscopic surgery, in and out of the hospital before noon, three little band aids and recovery time of a week.

Sure, tease me with an easy surgery my BRCA gene. Lure me into complacency since I have now reduced my breast cancer risk by 50%. My gynecologist had me see an oncologic gynecologist at Fox Chase. She suggested I start Tamoxifen prophylactically in 2006 for 5 years. Okay no biggie. It's only a pill, right? A teensy-weensy pill. Well that dot of a pill after a week left me feeling like an 80-year-old woman every morning. My bones hurt, my knees and hips were sore and it disrupted my GI tract. Fortunately that Fall I began having pain and itching in my right breast. Mammogram and ultrasounds showed nothing. Neither did the MRI. I visited my breast specialist who is also a high school friend. I knew he had my best interest at heart when he suggested I have a prophylactic bilateral mastectomy (PBM).

I was scheduled for my PBM on June 7, 2007. I was having an Alloderm one-step with 750 cc saline implants. All went well, at first. Every time they backed off the pain meds, my pain level elevated but when they increased the morphine, my oxygen levels dropped dramatically. I finally told them to just leave the morphine down and get me to my room. It was 11 PM and way past my bedtime!

That was a Monday. By Wednesday, the resident plastic surgeon (PS) noticed some necrotic tissue developing on my right breast. Thursday my PS took me back into the operating room and removed the tissue. Saturday I was back home with four drains that I named after the Beatles. Missing my precious morphine drip that kept me so happy. And the pathology showed they got clean margins of DCIS (Ductal Carcinoma In Situ), Stage 0 breast cancer, that nobody had anticipated. The sentinel nodes were also clear.

Now I realized how much having a shower meant to me. My husband, Larry, washed my hair and it was a "mechia," Yiddish for absolute nirvana. And one by one, my drains stopped draining and were removed by my PS. My best friend had arranged for other friends and relatives to bring in meals so Larry didn't have to worry about cooking. All he had to do was to take care of me.

My first of many setbacks began. Two weeks later I was back in the hospital with a 102 fever. They apparently suspected MRSA after testing for everything under the sun. They inserted a PICC line and sent me home. For three weeks I had a home infusion of Vancomycin for what turned out to be a double staph infection. What a treat! After that I was on two weeks of oral Clyndomycin, which I developed an allergy to. Fortunately, I was up, moving around and functioning.

My fourth and final drain that I named "Ringo" was with me for eight weeks total. We bonded so much that skin started to form around the tube. He wanted to stay, however he needed to leave. The PS tried a Betadine wash through Ringo. Nope. Infection got so bad that the body thought the saline implant was the intruder and tried to force it out. The fluid buildup was pushing the implant against the inside of the breast. A small hole opened up and I was leaking the fluid. My doctor tried sewing it up. The stitches did not hold and in

August I went in to have my left implant removed. I was so depressed. My family doctor put me on Cymbalta to help and I took Xanax to help me relax and sleep at night. Emotionally, I was a wreck!

After the infection was cleared up in January I had another surgery to have an expander inserted. "Rachel" my right foob (fake + boob) was missing her counterpart "Laverne" who came back for a return engagement in May 2008. Yay! I was healthy, cancer-free and glad to be here. In 2009 my PS stitched up one last revision. Then he asked, "How about nipples?" I had already gone out and purchased "Fipples," yup Fake + nipples. If I wanted to have headlights I could, but there was no way, shape or form I was having any more surgeries.

My 3-year follow-up appointment is scheduled for the end of May 2012. I am still getting breast checks with Dr. Mary Daly at FCCC. I am very involved with the local Philly FORCE Outreach Group (www.facebook.com/Philadelphia.PA.FORCE). I am giving back to a great group of people here at Beyond the Pink Moon. I am HERE!

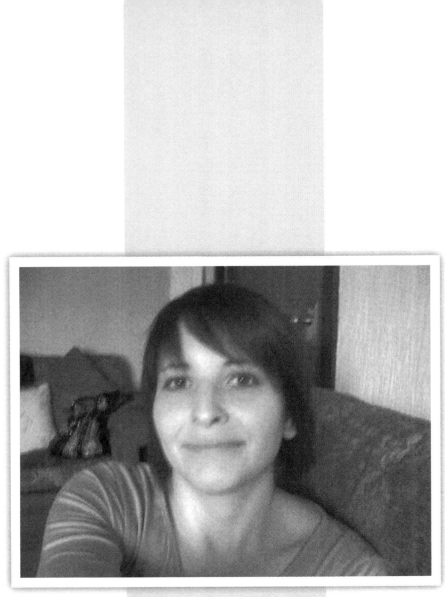

Christine Garrett

BRCA2 Survivor, 28
Belfast, NORTHERN IRELAND, UNITED KINGDOM

Taking Back My Life

I was 27 and worked in the intensive therapy unit (ICU) in a Belfast hospital. I had just come home from doing what we call a long day (8am-9pm) and sat down to have a chat with my mother. I stretched up and felt something strange on my breast. I showed my mum and she felt it as well. We both thought it was nothing, but decided it was best to err on the side of caution and have my General Practitioner (GP) check it.

The following day Mum and I planned to go to the Balmoral Show in Belfast. It's a big day for us country folk. We decided we should go ahead with our plans. In the meantime, I called my GP and got an appointment for later that day. We enjoyed our day and I went to the GP later that afternoon. She said it was nothing because of my age, but I demanded to be sent to a specialist, as there was a history of cancer in my family. Within a week I had an appointment at the Ulster Hospital for follow-up tests to be done.

I first met Mr. Kirk. He took a biopsy from the lump and sent it to pathology. In the meantime I had a lot of waiting around to do. I got a call for a mammogram and then more waiting. I went alone, as I was sure it was nothing. Three hours later I found myself waiting to be called into see Mr. Kirk for all the results. Looking back now I should have known there was something wrong, as I was the last person in the waiting area.

I was taken into a room with a lovely breast care nurse named Rosie and told that I had Grade 3 breast cancer. I just went blank. How the hell was I going to tell my parents, family, boyfriend and friends? There was no way this was happening to me. The calls I had to make after that news were the worst in my life. Telling everyone I still felt as if I was talking about a third party.

Within a month I had my lumpectomy. Chemo started four weeks after that and then radiotherapy. Chemo was awful, but it was only six treatments. I had to go every three weeks. The worst part was the sickness and the hair loss. Radiotherapy was a 'gift' compared to chemo.

I was then given the option to get genetic testing done, as there was a strong history of cancer on both sides of my family. So I took it. Deep down I kind of knew I had a genetic mutation.

This leads me to where I am today. I've been told I have the BRCA2 gene mutation and just don't know were to turn. But one thing is for sure, I'm not letting my family see me crumble again. I have decided to take back my life. I will have the prophylactic bilateral mastectomy (PBM) with reconstruction and will live my life empowered.

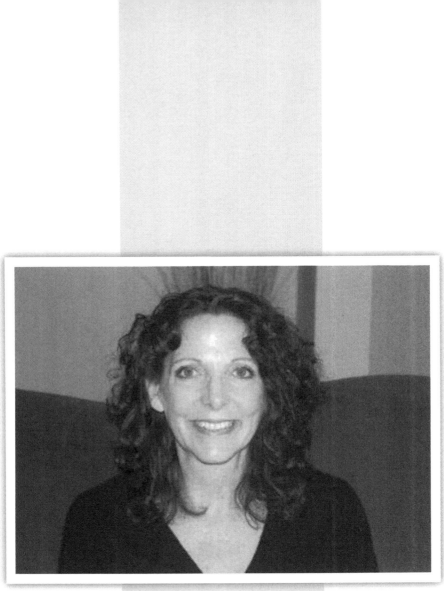

Susan Calhoun

BRCA1 Survivor, 53
Indianapolis, Indiana USA

Somewhere Over The Rainbow

In 1994 I sat for many days with my sister in the hospital as the breast cancer that had spread throughout her body had metastasized to her brain. We still shared good talks in her lucid moments and I will always cherish the time I spent with her. I would sing a song to her that was popular at the time by Joshua Kadison "Beautiful in my eyes". Because even with her bald little head and gaunt body ravaged by cancer, she was beautiful. At age 39 she succumbed to cancer, leaving four children under 13 years old.

Of course I had this superior attitude that my sister and I were so different. We were built differently, she all curvy and cute whereas I was tall and not so curvy. I ate very healthy, did not smoke, did not drink as she had, and exercised. In my mind I was not concerned that I would get cancer. No one before my sister had it. My mother had ten brothers and sisters and my father had two brothers and everyone lived cancer free to a ripe old age.

Nevertheless, I did begin getting yearly mammograms at age 34. Year after year they came back fine. Every once and awhile I would have to go back but it always turned out to be nothing until July 2010. They called me back in because the radiologist saw the faintest shadow. So faint that she did not think it was anything but called me to come in just in case. I happily went back in knowing that like all the other times I would be fine. The ultrasound showed more than a shadow. My breast doctor recommended a biopsy. As I have always requested honesty, she told me that it did not look good. She was right. She called and told me to come in that day because I had cancer. She said that with my sister's death and because I was also young (51) that she would like to test me for the BRCA gene mutation. I had three daughters and I wanted to know so she sent the blood work in that day. It came back positive for the BRCA1 gene mutation.

I met with oncologists and got second opinions about chemotherapy and was put on Cisplatin. My daughter Rachel took me to my first round of chemotherapy on August 9, 2010. It was such a comfort to have her there. I know the first round is usually the easiest, but I was so sick. My phone rang late the evening of the second day after my treatment. I saw that it was my daughter Kate calling. I just did not have the energy to even pick up the phone and figured I would call her back in the morning when I hopefully felt better. I wish I had picked up the phone. On August 11, 2010 my daughter, my baby Kate, after years of battling mental illness, took her life. There is a whole other story about life without Kate, but I won't write it here. What I will say is that the two most dreaded things in life, cancer and losing a child, had suddenly happened to me, and my mantra of "someone is always worse off than me, and have joy no matter what" was being severely tested.

Having to focus on chemo, staying healthy enough for treatments, plus continuing to work throughout my treatment took its toll. By the time my fourth treatment was nearing, I was having severe headaches so bad that I would bang my head against the wall... really. When I had my blood work done my creatinine levels were so high that my kidneys were in grave danger. I was immediately hospitalized. It was a horrible and very lonely ten days. I was so sick, but in the midst, when I thought I was going to lose it, a nurse came in and asked if she could pray with me. It was such a blessing and I knew I was going to survive however long I had to stay there. That was just one example of all the people whose paths crossed mine and made those five months bearable.

A few days before Thanksgiving I had my double mastectomy and came home and was cared for by my two daughters. They took such good care of me and even emptied my drains. Now that is certainly an act of love!!! It felt good to let go and let them take care of me. The worst was past, chemo was over, and my breasts were gone. I survived. My scars were now a part of me, my body changed, but I was okay. Things that used to matter (that should not have) just did not have any power over me. I had grown and it felt good.

My mother got tested for the gene and was negative. My father had already passed (suicide as well) but obviously it was he who had the gene. Strangely enough no one in his family had any cancer. My oldest brother tested positive and my other brother does not want to test. We assume my sister also had the gene. My oldest daughter has tested positive and is going to have a double mastectomy and her tubes taken out. She is such a strong woman who has courageously taken the bull by the horns and is getting the word out to others. My other daughter has not been tested but I hope she will soon.

Me, I am living life, two years a survivor, back to all the things I used to do, but with a more peaceful and settled attitude. It takes a lot to make me stress now. Like all the other women who have shared this gene I am changed forever, and grateful for the sisters I have out there who understand.

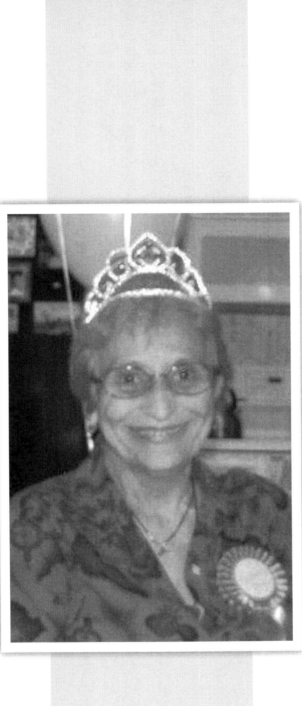

Rosie Goldstein

BRCA1 Ovarian Cancer Survivor, 68
Florida USA

My Journey With The Beast and BRCA1

I'm not really sure where to begin. For a couple of years I went to doctors complaining about bloating, constipation and pain. I was diagnosed with irritable bowl, colitis, and told to see a shrink.

Then on April 1, 2001 I moved to Florida and the bloating and pain got worse. Finally on Aug. 25, 2001 my BFF Dani called 911. The emergency room doctor removed over seven and a half liters of bloody fluid from my abdomen and told an attending nurse to call the gynecologist/oncologist. I had ovarian cancer. Everything became a blur for quite a while after that.

The next day I remember the gynecologist/oncologist coming into my room and telling me I had ovarian cancer. I asked. "Okay, what are we going to do about it?" He said, "I don't think you understand, YOU HAVE OVARIAN CANCER." Again I asked, "Okay, what are we going to do about it?" Then he came around to the side of my bed, took my hand and said, "Do you understand what I'm telling you?" I said, "Gilda Radner, I get it, now what the hell are we going to do about it!" Then he smiled at me and said, "I guess I've got a fighter on my hands!" I said, "You sure do!"

The next thing I knew I was in intensive care, I don't really know how long, but all major systems were shutting down. I don't remember much about that period except that on 9/11/01 I was scheduled for surgery. I woke up that morning to the news on CNN. Dani said, "Let's turn this off, it's a dumb movie." I told her I knew what it was and I wanted to know if there would be a world left for me to wake up to after surgery. She tried to shield me. I'm not easy to fool!

When I was recovered enough from the surgery to go home, I woke up one morning and could not move. My back and legs were in excruciating pain. My doctor ordered an MRI. I had herniated a disc in my back in my sleep.

He scheduled me to see a neurosurgeon just before Christmas. I was medicated; the IVs were in as I waited for the surgeon to come by. When he walked in with my chart in his hand he looked at me, saw my bald head, stopped and said, "Who is your doctor?" I told him and he said, "You have cancer I'm not touching you." He turned around and walked out leaving the anesthesiologist, the nurses and me with our mouths hanging open. The nurses asked, "What do we do now?" The anesthesiologist said, "I'll give her the reversal drugs and have her taken back up to her room."

I finally scheduled someone to operate on my back after the holiday. It was too late. The nerve damage was done and unable to be repaired. The surgeon that walked out on me left the area for parts unknown.

I immediately signed up for a cancer study after my surgery. Without getting my notebooks out, I went through I don't know how many chemos. I was lucky. I went into remission for two months shy of six years. Then it came back with a vengeance! Six tumors spread to the lymph nodes. Another study, lots of chemo and my PET scan finally came back clear. Three months later it came back again with four tumors and a few positive nodes. No biggie! I'm ready to get this party rolling and show the beast who's the boss once and for all!

PREVIVORS

Individuals who are survivors of a predisposition to cancer but who haven't had the disease. This group includes people who carry a hereditary mutation, a family history of cancer, or some other predisposing factor.

Melissa Johnson Voight

BRCA1 Previvor, 44
Newport News, Virginia USA

Beauty From Ashes

In November 2009 I received a phone call from one of my family members informing me that my cousin, Karen, was diagnosed with a very aggressive form of breast cancer. Through her blood work and tests, she found out that she carried the same BRCA1 gene mutation that our paternal grandmother had. She passed away when she was only 41 years young. We also found out that my dad and both of his brothers were also positive for the BRCA1 mutation. My cousin's oncologist suggested that all of the cousins (boys and girls) be tested to see if we also carried the gene.

My sister, Kim, wasted no time and made an appointment for both of us. On March 3, 2010 we arrived at Walter Reed Hospital, in Gloucester, VA. We had our blood drawn to be tested and they gave us an estimated waiting time of two weeks for the results to return. During this time, I kept asking myself, "What if"? What if the result comes back that I am positive for this genetic mutation? If it came back that I was a carrier, I knew what choice I would ultimately make for myself. Again I asked, "What if I do have this?" I heard God speak to me within my soul," I will make beauty from ashes." I simply had to TRUST Him and take His hand. I knew right then, in my heart, what my result was going be. God was preparing me for a journey with Him.

Two weeks came and went and we received a call from my oncologist. Trying to stay hopeful, but knowing in my heart what I was going to hear, I entered the waiting room with my sister. My name was called and my sister and I were led into a room. The oncologist entered. My hands were sweating and my heart was racing. She looked at my sister and said, "You do NOT have the gene mutation." Then she turned and looked at me and said, "But you do." That gut feeling I had been experiencing for two weeks was now a reality. There was no longer the question of "what if"... but, "what now?" There it was, in black and white, "Positive for Deleterious Genetic Mutation." The oncologist told me that I had an 87% chance of getting breast cancer. I could lower that risk to 50% by having a Bilateral Salpingo Oophorectomy (removal of both ovaries and fallopian tubes also known as a BSO) or lower it further to 3% by also having a prophylactic bilateral mastectomy (PBM). I turned and looked at my sister, and said, "It's okay ~ It's going to be okay!" As we left the office, my sister called my mom and gave her the results of our tests. My mom had been so certain that we would both be negative for the gene, but we assured her that I was going to be alright and that I knew what I had to do in order to be safe, have hope and a future.

I was 41, the same age as my dad's mom, who passed away from this very gene. Married with two children. I knew what I had to do. I looked at it as a blessing, a gift from God, to have the knowledge of what was waiting for me down the road, before it even happened.

This isn't a matter of "if" breast cancer was going to touch my life, but a matter of "when." I didn't want to keep looking over my shoulder waiting for the ball to drop. I wanted to be here with my family and the ones I dearly love.

I texted Karen to let her know that I also tested positive for the BRCA1 mutation. Karen encouraged me to have the prophylactic surgeries. She sympathized with me that I was going to have to do this. I felt guilty knowing that Karen was fighting for her life. However her diagnosis gave me, as well as other family members, a chance to live. How could I not take this gift? As this all unfolded, it was like opening Pandora's box. One by one my whole family tested. Some results were positive for the gene mutation while others tested negative. We rejoiced in the negative tests results and comforted those who tested positive.

In the days following the test results, I made a lot of phone calls and scheduled appointments to determine which doctors I would use to perform my surgeries. I had one appointment after another. For someone who hated going to the doctors, I was having my fair share of them. I had an MRI, blood work, and a mammogram, all prior to my surgeries. I also met with a surgical oncologist and a plastic surgeon. On March 30th, 2010, I had a BSO, performed by my gynecologist. A week later, the hot flashes began. Only one of the side affects to having my ovaries removed. And on May 7th, 2010, I had a PBM, with immediate reconstruction.

When I woke up after my surgery, I was wearing a tightly fitted sports bra, with drainage tubes under both sides of my arms. The tubes drained excess fluid from my chest. I had expanders where my breasts use to be. My plastic surgeon was able to add 125cc of saline in my expanders, to begin my reconstruction. I was able to return home the following day.

A week later I returned to my plastic surgeon to have the drains removed. Two weeks later they began injecting saline into the expanders. This was stretching the skin to make room for the implants, which would be exchanged on a later date. I went back every week, for the next four weeks for saline injections. After I reached a total of 275 ccs, I waited for two months. On August 15, 2010, I had the expanders removed and the gummy bear implants fitted. I was glad to finally be rid of the solid rock expanders. My plastic surgeon compared the transfer from expander to implant, to that of taking off stiletto heels and putting on slippers. I felt like a million bucks!

After having the necessary procedures to lower my ovarian and breast cancer risks, I opted to do nipple reconstruction. This was done under local anesthesia in October 2010. It was fairly quick and simple. But days after the procedure the left nipple began to turn dark. I called the on call doctor who requested I come in the next day. My plastic surgeon thought it looked like it was going recover and heal, and sent me home to keep an eye on it. The next day it was darker than the day before. It wasn't looking good and I began fearing the worst. Then over the weekend it turned black and died. I was horrified and cried uncontrollably. Everything had gone so well, prior to this procedure, and then this! I questioned God's promises that everything was going to be alright. "You told me everything was going to be okay?" Why this? Why now?" Still God told me to trust Him, and that it was all going to be okay... we were just taking a slight detour, in order for Him to spend more time growing me spiritually. I will admit, I felt myself wanting to run ahead of Him, as soon as I saw the light at the end of this journey. Instead of walking with Him...

beside Him... I was leaving Him behind and expecting Him to keep up with me. That's not how it was meant to be. Still God told me to trust Him, so the journey continued.

When I returned back to my plastic surgeon's office he set up an appointment for me to have the dead tissue removed. Weeks later we rescheduled another appointment to remake another nipple. My surgeon gave me a 98% chance of it surviving and it did. A few months later the left nipple began to flatten out. At this point I wasn't sure what to do next. I was told that there was another option, 3-D tattooing. Wow!! I thought that sounded interesting. At this point what did I have to lose? In March 2011 I went to the surgeon's cosmetic technician and began the process. After many months and five appointments it was done!

I can finally say I am very pleased with the outcome of my journey! I praise God for sustaining me through it all. It wasn't always easy or what I expected, but the bottom line is that I am alive and well. It has been a full two years of testing, appointments, doctor's visits, surgeries, procedures, and ups and downs. But I can't complain. We are blessed! We live in a time where we can be tested for these genetic mutations. We have a choice! My choice was to take the gift of extending my life. Sure I had to make a radical decision, but I can be here with my loved ones. BRCA1 testing saved my life. Had it not been for Karen's journey, cancer could have touched any one of my family member's lives. I don't want Karen's fight to be wasted. We need to educate our family members of their risks and encourage them to take action. Karen's journey will not be in vain. She gave us a gift. She would want us to take that gift and run with it, looking forward confident and empowered.

Jeremiah 29:11 says,

"For I know the plans I have for you, "declares the Lord," plans to prosper you and not to harm you, plans to give you a hope and a future."

As I look back over the past year, I am truly amazed at God's love and tender mercy. His grace is truly sufficient, and His faithfulness is true! God always keeps His promises ~ always!

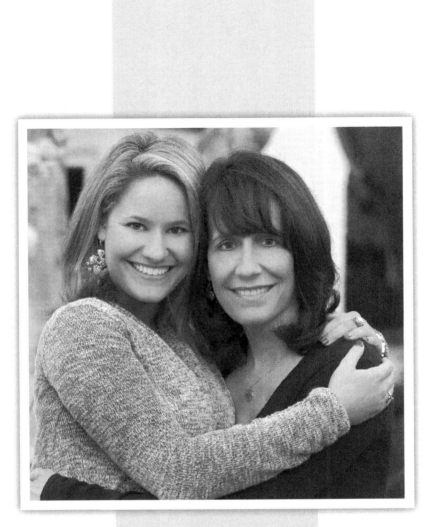

Ally Bianchina Durlester with her mother, Nicki Boscia Durlester

Ally Bianchina Durlester

BRCA2 Previvor, 25
Los Angeles, California USA

Bianchina's Granddaughter

I always smile. I am a happy person. I lived a charmed life until October 2010 when I tested positive for the BRCA2 mutation. I was 23 years old.

Although the BRCA gene hid in the shadows of my life, it was never at the forefront. For as long as I can remember my mom has shared vivid tales about her big Italian family. Most of the stories were light-hearted and painted pictures of the happy childhood she had growing up in Pennsylvania. She loved to tell me about the delicious feasts my grandmother, Bianchina, cooked. Her favorite memories are of Christmas Eve, a tradition we still carry on in our home. But, I also see the sadness in my mom's eyes when she speaks about her mother, the grandmother I never had the chance to meet. She passed away long before I was born, at the age of 58, from fallopian tube cancer. More than a decade earlier she had survived breast cancer. Six of my grandmother's seven sisters also had breast or ovarian cancer. It was a staggering family history of malignancy and loss that my mom rarely talked about it. It all came bubbling to the surface in 2009 when my mother was diagnosed with breast cancer. I was a junior in college. Suddenly everything became real. It wasn't just family folklore anymore. My grandmother, Bianchina, whose name I share, left a beautiful legacy and fond memories that will be passed down through the generations. She also unknowingly passed down the BRCA2 gene mutation.

It was a normal weekday in October 2010. I was home cleaning out my closet when my cell phone rang. My mother, who was sitting on my bed watching, answered it for me. It was her breast surgeon, Dr. Kristi Funk, calling with my BRCA test result. With hesitation she handed me the phone. Dr. Funk matter-of-factly said, "Ally you tested positive for the BRCA2 mutation. Let's set up a time for you to come into the office so we can discuss what this means and what your options are." In a bubbly and perky tone I responded, "Sounds good. I will call you in a few days to schedule an appointment." SOUNDS GOOD? Honestly, who would say that when they have just been told they carry a genetic mutation that will increase their lifetime risk of breast cancer to 85% and ovarian cancer to 54%? When I look back on that day over two years ago I realize I was in shock. Being told I had the BRCA2 mutation felt like I had been shot in the stomach. My mother was so upset that I didn't have a second to react. I felt so badly for her. I knew she felt responsible.

For the first couple of months I swept my feelings under the carpet. My mother had just published her memoir about her breast cancer journey and we were busy doing interviews and signings for Beyond the Pink Moon. I had taken a leave of absence from my job to help her with her book tour. My mother kept asking me if I was alright and I continued to reassure her it was no big deal. I always smile, remember?

Shortly after finding out my BRCA test result I accompanied my mother to a CNN interview. I wasn't supposed to be on camera that day. When the broadcaster asked if I had been tested for the gene I blurted out I was positive for the BRCA2 mutation. The broadcaster wanted to break the news on camera. Suddenly I was the star attraction. Caught up in the moment I had no time to think about my feelings. So there I was on camera sharing my secret with the world without having time to digest it myself.

The truth is I hid my feelings because I did not want my parents to worry about me. And the last thing I wanted was to have my mom feeling guilty about passing down the gene. It wasn't her fault. It wasn't anyone's fault. She had been opposed to me testing for the gene. She didn't think I was ready to deal with a potential positive result and all of the ramifications from that. She was right. I wasn't emotionally prepared. At the beginning of the New Year in 2011 I had a breakdown and for most of that year I felt lost. I suffered from severe anxiety for the first time in my life. I was unable to wrap my head around the news that my breasts and ovaries were ticking time bombs. Overwhelmed does not even begin to describe how I felt. I did not want to talk about it or make any decisions about prophylactic surgeries. I needed time to think it through. I wasn't smiling anymore. I needed help to face the thought of my newfound mortality. It took months of therapy and the love and support of my parents to finally breathe again and make decisions that were right for me.

I have chosen to practice active surveillance with Dr. Funk as my head coach. I know I am in the best of hands with her. Every six months I have a clinical breast exam, staggering my tests including mammogram, ultrasound and MRI. Although I have minimal risk of breast cancer from the BRCA2 mutation prior to age 30, I am planning on having my prophylactic bilateral mastectomy in 2013 at the age of 26. I have heard of a few cases of BRCA2 women who were diagnosed with breast cancer in their twenties. I don't want to tempt fate for too long. My risk for ovarian cancer kicks in later in my 30s. My plan is to have my ovaries removed by the time I'm 35. For now, I have six-month check-ups with my gynecologist who performs a transvaginal ultrasound and CA-125 blood test.

Two years later and I am still standing, stronger than ever. I only have one life to live and I will not allow the BRCA2 gene mutation to ruin the rest of mine. This experience has taught me that all human beings cope with adversity and difficult situations differently. There is no right or wrong way to react to something. Finding out I had the BRCA2 gene mutation was a blow, but it didn't knock me out. We have a choice with everything in life. We can chose to sink into a lifetime of fear and anxiety or we can dig down deep and Push On Try Again. POTA has always been my motto, one that I will continue to embrace throughout my life.

Having the BRCA2 mutation has opened my eyes and has helped me to identify a new path in my life. I have accepted my reality and refuse to be bitter about it. I have learned my lessons and I am enriched for it. I always smile. I am a happy person. This *is* who I am.

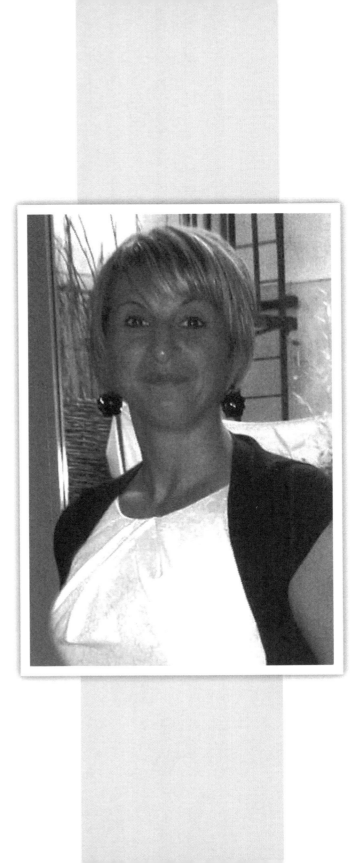

Brenda K. Ritzco

BRCA2 Previvor, 40
Dallas, Texas USA

Running with the Enemy

"We're surrounded. That simplifies the problem..." Chesty Puller

Write my story... not sure I have one. It's more of a collection of rambling thoughts, questions and fears scribbled on post-its and in notebooks. I am the Warrior Queen's sister and since I know the enemy, many cannot understand the choices I have made. You might not like the things I have to say, but this is my story.

I have read hundreds of accounts of prophylactic surgeries from women asking for prayers before reconstruction or when things go wrong because of complications. I have also read the countless journeys of young women forced into premature menopause from prophylactic oophorectomies. I cannot relate to any of it.

I believe there are a lot of young women thinking the same way I do, but not courageous enough to say it out loud. I do not want prophylactic surgery. When I take my clothes off I want nipples I can feel and a wet vagina. Yep, I said it. Women really don't talk about it, but I want to enjoy myself. I don't want tattooed nipples on perfectly perky breasts. It's not just about the physical. I will be miserable if I alter myself. It will suffocate my spirit and that is something I cannot live with.

I believe a lot of women think about their bodies the way I do. They want their own functional feminine parts. They may not, however, have the courage to say it in a climate where the majority of women with the BRCA mutation seem to be having prophylactic surgeries. I know I have BRCA bomb boobs. It doesn't mean I can't like them. I think women say boobs are overrated or their boobs don't define them out of fear, guilt, or their way of coping with their loss. I get that. Cancer is all around them. But, it's okay to love your body with or without boobs, foobs, or BRCA bombs. Some people think I would rather get cancer by my decision to forego a preemptive strike. I find that ignorant. Why would I want cancer?

Sun Tzu Art of War...Know Thyself to Know Thy Enemy.... "If you know your enemies and know yourself, you can win hundreds of battles without a single loss." The old saying, keep your friends close and your enemies closer. I choose to live with my enemy.

In April 2010, I went to a genetic counselor after my younger sister, Barbara (the Warrior Queen), was diagnosed with Stage III breast cancer at 36. Genetic testing revealed she had the BRCA2 mutation. There was a 50/50 chance I would also inherit the mutation. BINGO!! I won the lottery. I was also a BRCA2 mutant. Not happy about it... just my sarcasm and sick humor.

Later we would find out that my first cousin Linda, my paternal Uncle Johnny's daughter, was diagnosed with breast cancer at 33. She was also BRCA2 positive. We never thought anything of it. We assumed it came from her mother's side of the family. We didn't list it in our medical history or even think about breast cancer. Boy were we ever wrong!!!

Many families with the BRCA mutation have generational stories of breast and ovarian cancers along with other malignancies linked to the gene mutations. Our family did not know until now that our fathers passed down the mutation in our genes. My dad had three girls including my younger sisters Tammy, Barbara, and me. My Uncle Johnny had one child, his daughter Linda. We each had a 50/50 chance of inheriting the genetic mutation. We all lost the coin toss in our family. Lucky SOBs we are. Wish we could play those odds in Vegas. Unfortunately we were blindsided when my sister Barb and cousin Linda were both diagnosed with Stage III breast cancer. Thankfully my sister Tammy and I are both previvors. Tammy quickly chose to have prophylactic surgeries. She was married with three beautiful daughters and wanted to be there for them and not have to deal with the anxiety of what if.

When I received my BRCA result my genetic counselor did a poor job of explaining what I should do next. She assumed because my sister was recently diagnosed with breast cancer that I knew what to do or what doctors to meet with, but I had no clue. I sank into months of depression.

After receiving my results I submerged myself in breast cancer groups, books, FORCE and anything I could gain information on BRCA mutations. So submerged, I drowned. I cried every day for months sometimes five or six times a day. I must have felt my breasts ten times a day, paranoid I would find a lump. I cried at work. If people asked about my sister, I cried. I talked to whoever would listen.

At the time I was living in Texas and had no family near me. Since my sister was battling breast cancer the family focus was on her. I am thankful for my co-workers in Dallas. They must have been so tired of me talking about whether or not I should remove my breasts, but they continued to listen and supported me. I was consumed with what decisions I should make. I didn't want to be haunted by the wrong choice. If I choose surveillance and got cancer people would say that I knew and did nothing to stop it.

I decided to see a therapist to gain the advice and counsel of a professional, someone neutral and unbiased. At first I was skeptical, but soon looked forward to my sessions. I would go right after work to her office, take my shoes off and plop down on her couch. It felt so good to purge everything in my head. I felt clearer and able to make better decisions. My therapist told me I was grieving. This puzzled me since no one had died. She explained loss without death to me. It all made sense. I was grieving for my sisters and my nieces and the thought of removing my healthy breasts and ovaries. I was consumed with worry about my family and the enemy living with us. While obsessing about my options I chose to begin active surveillance. A friend wisely told me, "Brenda make a decision and own it."

Surveillance

I scheduled all my doctor appointments. The bills started piling up fast. Even though I had insurance I had a $1,500 deductible to meet and I had a $50 co-pay every time I saw a specialist. My insurance coverage maxed out at 80/20.

My first mammogram resulted in a call back within 24 hours. They needed more pictures of my right breast, which thankfully showed there wasn't anything there. In February I decided to have a breast MRI since I wasn't certain about having a prophylactic bilateral mastectomy (PBM) during the summer. I had my MRI in the morning before work and received a phone call an hour after I left the imaging center. I knew it couldn't be good so I didn't answer the phone. I went in my office, closed the door and listened to the voicemail. They saw something in my left breast and wanted me to come back for an ultrasound. When I called to schedule the appointment the nurse said it was actually my right breast that needed an ultrasound and possible biopsy. I went into a panic. WTF! I had three mammograms in the last year and none of this was seen. Where did this come from so fast? I thought it had to be cancer since typically BRCA positive cancer is more aggressive due to the fact that a mutation carrier lacks one tumor suppressor gene. Then I thought about the melanoma I was diagnosed with in 2005. The doctor said mine was the most aggressive type.

I scheduled my appointment for the ultrasound and possible biopsy the next morning. I asked the ultrasound tech which breast they were looking at since both were questionable. She said the right breast since the left one had just a cyst. Of course I overreacted to "just a cyst." I just spent months reading breast cancer horror stories. After asking the tech what seemed like a thousand questions, I felt at ease that it was just a cyst in my left breast. The tech moved the ultrasound wand over my right breast for what seemed like an hour trying to locate what they saw on the MRI. The radiologist did the same thing. It was so nerve-racking. I kept thinking this is it. A year to date after my sister's diagnosis here comes mine. The doctor finally located the mass. It was the size of a pea. She said it was far behind my nipple near my chest wall. I asked her why I never felt it. She said not even a clinical breast exam would have found it. I was getting very anxious and sweat was pouring out of me, soaking the sheet covering me. The doctor told me she did not feel comfortable doing the biopsy guided by the ultrasound. She wanted to do an MRI guided core biopsy. I had no idea what this entailed. I was told to get dressed because they had to get approval from my insurance company. I waited for hours before I was finally called back in. They explained the procedure, but I had no idea how painful it would be. I was face down in the MRI, my breast smashed tight, while they punctured my breast with a needle the size of a pen. It felt like it was poking through the other side. I was screaming. They called another tech in to assist. This is where the bottom fell out for me. The reality of being BRCA2 finally hit home. I was crying so hard I thought I was going to drown in my tears. It was horrible. I was there by myself because I didn't think I needed help. They put a clip in my breast where the mass was so they could easily find it in the future. Thank God it was a benign fibroadenoma. As crazy as it sounds that moment of panic and freak-out set me free. It cleared my head of fears. I embraced my enemy and knew I was strong enough to choose surveillance and whatever my future holds. Some say I'm choosing cancer if I don't remove my breasts. I believe I am choosing life.

Faith

As I struggled with my decision to remove my breasts and ovaries my wonderful friends and their faith in God kept me strong. Sometimes I find it perplexing when people ask for prayers and talk about faith. Why not leave all of this in God's hands then? Maybe my faith is stronger or maybe I'm a fool. Do I put science before faith or faith before science? It's a conundrum to me.

In my darkest moments I struggled with the best decisions or right choices for myself. I listened to everyone I talked to and carefully considered it all. I had many interesting conversations with a teacher who was also a minister. He purchased a book for me about generational curses, a very interesting read and faith perspective. My conversations with him were comforting. I grew up in the Catholic Church and found Catholicism very disappointing. In church and Sunday school I learned very little about the bible. My conversations with coworkers were comforting and their connections to church and God were inspiring to me. I didn't pray or go to church, but I always welcomed their conversations because they were enlightening and educational.

More and more I meet women who choose prophylactic surgeries who look down on women who choose active surveillance. No one has a crystal ball about the future. People say you only live once, which is not true. You die once. You live everyday. And I am living.

It may sound crazy and naïve knowing my risks, but I feel like I'm going to be okay. If I get cancer people will say I was a fool, but if I don't maybe my body will offer up some secrets as to why I didn't get cancer and why my sister and cousin did. My mind is at ease and I'm no longer stressed out everyday. Even my breast surgeon/oncologist said if I am not mentally ready it would not be healthy for me to have prophylactic surgeries. Hearing that was comforting to me, however I chose to keep an appointment with a plastic surgeon I had heard speak at a hereditary breast and ovarian conference in Dallas. I thought he would be a good match for me. When I went for my consultation it was disappointing to me. The doctor did not explain what to expect with regards to the surgery. My meeting with him confirmed what I had tortured myself about for a year. I was keeping my breast and ovaries and I was comfortable with that decision.

The thought of all the surgeries exhausted me. I think what bothers me the most about choosing surveillance is if I do get cancer people will say I told you so. I come from a long line of stubborn fighters on both sides of my family. I will not live in fear or allow my life to be governed by what ifs. The possibility does not scare me because I have accepted it. I believe because the choice to have prophylactic surgeries was so hard to make, it wasn't the right one for me. All I know for certain is that there are no guarantees in life and I'm going to live. Being a mutant brought out my competitive side. I am a walking risk so why not take the risks I want to. I started running again and fell in love with Obstacle Racing. I have become pretty good for my age. So for now I will be running with the enemy, keeping close tabs on him.

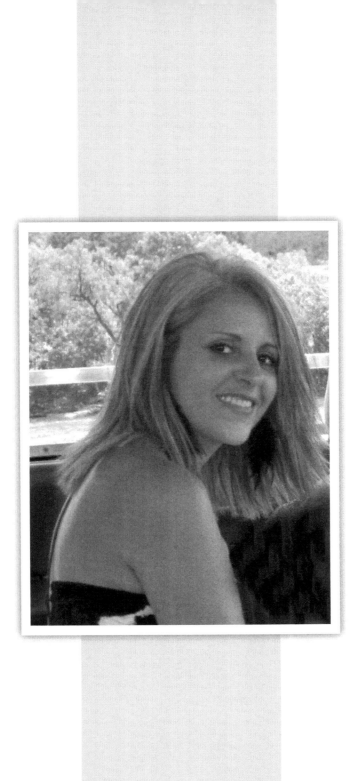

Teri Smieja

BRCA1 Previvor, 42
Alexandria, Virginia USA

The Gift of Life

It may seem weird for a woman who has never had breast or ovarian cancer to think about it as much as I do. In fact, I thought about it so much I chose to have a prophylactic (refers to the removal of healthy tissue and fat) hysterectomy and bilateral salpingo oopherectomy (BSO) in October 2009, just a few days before my 39th birthday. I also had both of my breasts removed during a prophylactic bilateral mastectomy (PBM) in February 2010.

While I don't have breast or ovarian cancer, I do have a genetic mutation of my BRCA1 gene, which makes my risk of getting breast cancer up to 87% and my ovarian cancer risk up to 44% over my lifetime. The average woman has an 8% chance. While science has come a long way, at this point in time, the best option for a woman with this mutation to avoid getting breast or ovarian cancer is to have her breasts and ovaries removed before the cancer strikes. In other words, the best way to fight cancer for us is to not get it in the first place, by removing our healthy breasts and ovaries.

When I first found out about my mutation I was thrown into a world of confusion and fear. Not only was my risk of cancer high but I also learned that diligent surveillance would likely not be a good enough option for me. The type of cancer associated with BRCA mutations is very aggressive and reoccurrences of breast cancer are high. I could battle and beat breast cancer, only to have it come after me again and again. The reason the cancer acts so aggressively on those of us with mutated genes is because we are missing our tumor suppressors. Our bodies are missing (in our DNA) the natural ability to protect itself against these types of cancer.

I have a lovely family including a husband and two sons. Of course the idea of going through with these surgeries scared me senseless, but my fear of getting and dying of breast and/or ovarian cancer scared me even more. I value my life more than my body parts. My older son, Steven, is a sophomore in college. My younger son, Brady, is just three years old. What message would it convey to my sons if I decided that I couldn't go through with the surgeries, if I just couldn't make myself part with my breasts and reproductive organs, and ended up with breast cancer? Wouldn't that teach them to value our outside appearance more than our life? What of my toddler who has no understanding of what is going on? How would my husband explain to our young son that his Mommy died because she was too afraid to take the best preventative steps that are available at this time?

As fearful as I was of having my breasts cut off, and my repro-ductive organs scooped out, I was so much more fearful of the alternative. I began to see the knowledge of my BRCA1 mutation as a gift rather than a curse. There is no denying the choices previvors like myself have to make are incredibly hard, but at least, if we take action soon enough, we do have a choice – something many of our relatives and friends didn't have. We have the ability to be pro-active in our battle rather than to sit around waiting for cancer to strike. I feel empowered, blessed and brave. Yes, brave, because while at times my insides may shake with fear, I was selfless enough to do what I needed to do, to be around for my family.

For me, worrying only about myself and my struggles through the land of living with a deleted area on my DNA wasn't enough. I found myself with so much empathy for other BRCA positive women forced to make these choices. Men can and do get this mutation as well, but the implications for women are more obvious, and come with a solution. A difficult solution, but a solution nevertheless. Initially I started blogging as a way to help myself make sense of all the fear and decisions that were suddenly placed before me. It didn't take long for me to see that by sharing openly of myself that it was helpful to other women going through the same thing. My blog, Teri's Blip in the Universe, is something I created that I'm incredibly proud of. To find a way to take an absolutely terrifying situation and turn it into something good and positive has been life changing for me. Later, when I co-created the BRCA Sisterhood group on Facebook with my good friend, Karen Malkin-Lazavoritz, my pride grew by leaps and bounds. To bring so many people together in a social environment that many of us use daily has been amazing.

Since I found out about my BRCA1 positive status I've had a chance to hear a lot of stories from others with the BRCA mutation, along with those with unknown mutations, or simply a family history laced with breast cancer, who decide to be proactive – who decide to be previvors.

The point is, I have a BRCA mutation, but it doesn't have to own me, it doesn't have to be an automatic death sentence. The cliché that knowledge is power may be overused (it's a cliché for a reason, right?), but few others fit better. Genetic testing gives us knowledge of a very probable cancer diagnosis and the ability to be proactive in our fight – which is truly the gift of life.

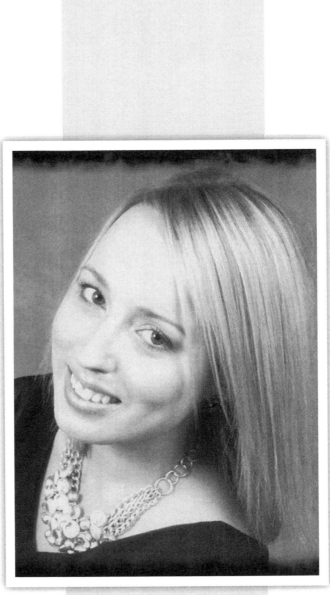

Carly Surber

BRCA1 Previvor, 24
San Diego, California USA

Choices.

"All men and women are born, live, suffer and die; what distinguishes us one from another are our dreams, whether they be dreams about worldly or unworldly things, and what we do to make them come about... We do not choose to be born. We do not choose our parents. We do not choose our historical epoch, the country of our birth, or the immediate circumstances of our upbringing. We do not, most of us, choose to die; nor do we choose the time and conditions of our death. But within this realm of choicelessness, we do choose how we live." Joseph Epstein

December 24, 2007.

It was a Christmas Eve spent much like other holidays in our house. It was only our immediate family: my parents, my brother, and myself relaxing and enjoying each other's company, but it felt different. I could not quite figure out why but something seemed off. My mom got up and went back to her bedroom and took my dad with her. I remember thinking how strange that was. We are a very open family, we rarely keep secrets from each other, but I brushed it off since it was Christmas Eve; maybe they were talking about gifts. Those pleasant thoughts were quickly replaced by stomach-churning emotions.

My mom told my older brother and I to come back to her room. We walked down the hallway and into their bedroom and that is when she told us. My mom informed us that she had a mammogram and they called her to schedule a biopsy. In her typical, straightforward manner, she told us that she had a feeling that it was cancer and that we should be prepared. I remember nothing else about Christmas that year. I cannot tell you about the gifts that were exchanged nor could I tell you what we ate for Christmas dinner. Four days later, she received the results. My mom, at the age of 54, had Stage III breast cancer and what was thought to be Stage IV at other times. It was very aggressive and likely deadly. That same day, not knowing what to do but wanting to show her support, I got a tattoo on my ribs of a pink breast cancer ribbon.

A brief history: As I grew up my maternal grandmother, DiDi to most but "Grandmère" to me, was always around. She lived in Los Angeles and we would visit often. When I was about 13 and as she aged, she moved into our house with us in San Diego. I always knew that she did not have breasts. I remember being very young and seeing her prosthetic breasts on her nightstand and I never asked questions. In my innocence and naivety, I thought that all older women lost their breasts. It was only later that I learned that she had been diagnosed with breast cancer on two different occasions and survived when the odds were heavily weighed against her. It was not until November 1, 2011 that she passed away at the age of 89 of an illness unrelated to cancer. I also learned that my great-grandmother had passed away from ovarian cancer at a relatively young age. Of the 18 closest relatives on my mother's side of the family, including my mother and myself, 8 tested positive for BRCA and 6 of those 8 women have had cancer. The women who have already passed away were not tested but are assumed to have been BRCA positive.

January 30, 2008.

My mom underwent a bilateral mastectomy. She and her doctors had decided to remove both breasts due to our strong family history and the likelihood of a recurrence. The surgery went well and she was incredibly tough.

About two weeks after her surgery she returned to work. Shortly after she began chemotherapy. I went to every chemotherapy appointment with her except for one because I had the flu. It was a very special time for me and I learned so much about my mom. I could tell that she was tired; I could tell that she was sick; but not once did she show fear. The grace that she exuded throughout her battle against cancer is something that I will never forget. I will also never forget the love that my dad showed for my mom. My dad acted in the most unconditionally loving manner I have ever witnessed. They both taught me quite a bit during such an emotional time.

In talking to my mom after her diagnosis she told me that she was not scared, she was at peace with her diagnosis and wanted to enjoy the time that she had in case she did not survive. She told me that she always had a feeling that she would one day be diagnosed with breast cancer. Little did she know, it was in her genes. After her diagnosis, her doctor informed her of the BRCA1 and BRCA2 gene mutations. We were previously unaware that such a thing existed.

She was tested and her results came back: She was positive for a genetic mutation referred to as BRCA1.

April 15, 2008.

My mom was in the midst of what I called a battle and what she called just another "thing" she had to deal with; she never felt as though she was fighting. I was 19 years old and in my second year of undergraduate studies. We decided to talk to a genetic counselor. Our genetic counselor charted our family history with all of the occurrences of breast and ovarian cancer and who had tested positive for the gene mutation. After seeing it written on paper, it became obvious to me that I could actually test positive for the gene mutation. A substantial number of women on the maternal side of my family were in fact BRCA1 positive. While not all had cancer, the risk was there. Of the 18 closest relatives on the maternal side of my family, eight women had tested positive for BRCA1gene mutation and six of those eight had at one point had cancer. The women who had died of female cancers are also assumed to have been BRCA1 positive. So with an incredible number of women in my family having tested positive for the genetic mutation and with a 50% chance of having the mutation myself, I sat in the lab and gave one small tube of blood and returned home to wait for the results.

April 30, 2008.

After 15 days I found myself, at 19 years old, sitting in a room at the hospital with my mom and our genetic counselor awaiting the verdict. During the two weeks I was waiting for the results, I had begun to research what it would mean for my future should I test positive. I knew that I had a 50% chance of having the mutation and

I knew that should I test positive, I would have to make big decisions regarding my future. I remember sitting in the room with my mom and she kept telling me "well, maybe you'll be negative". I had a feeling I would not be receiving such news. Our genetic counselor entered the room, opened up a purple folder that contained the test results, and informed me that I tested positive for a genetic mutation: "POSITIVE FOR A DELETERIOUS MUTATION" to be exact. I was now labeled as BRCA1 positive. She gave me numerous pieces of literature and discussed steps that I could take to reduce my risk. I really cannot remember anything she said in the moments immediately following the news, other than agreeing that I would receive special breast MRIs and regular clinical breast exams to make sure that if any cancer did develop, it would be caught at an early stage. I also began seeing a gynecological oncologist to discuss my increased risk for ovarian cancer. After many appointments with many doctors, I felt confident that we had implemented the best surveillance plan for me. At 19, I did not feel that surgical options were something that I would be willing to explore.

In the following years, my mom recovered from her chemo, her hair grew back, and regained her strength. I had since graduated with my bachelor's degree and had been admitted to law school in San Diego.

January 9, 2012.

Almost four years after my mom's mastectomy, at the age of 23, I informed my mom, my dad, and my boyfriend that I wanted to take action. Not only did I spend those four years creating memories, and doing all of the things that I wanted to do, I spent a lot of time researching the risks that I faced as a BRCA1 positive woman. I spoke with many women in the same position as I. And after four long years of deliberation I had enough. Midway through my first year of law school, I decided that I would have a prophylactic skin-sparing bilateral mastectomy. Looking back, I do not think that my parents believed me. I think that they may have thought that this was another phase and that I would change my mind. My mom, my Grandmère, and many other women before me did not have a choice whether or not to get breast cancer. The knowledge that I was given by having genetic testing was a gift. It empowered me. It gave me a choice.

I scheduled a consultation with a breast surgeon and met with him. It was an awful experience. I spoke to him about my fears and that I wanted to have this done so that I would never have to face what the women before me in my family had faced. There I sat, 23 years old, discussing the possibility of making a life-changing decision and this doctor did not look me in the eyes once. He was very cold and made me feel extremely uncomfortable. I left that appointment upset and doubting my decision to pursue this surgery.

Next I met with a plastic surgeon. This was a completely different experience. He made me feel extremely comfortable. He spent quite a lot of time explaining the reconstruction process, which was im-portant to me because my mom did not undergo reconstruction so my knowledge was lacking. He answered all of my questions and really put me at ease. I asked people that worked at the same hospital about him and they said he was the best. He referred me to a female doctor who I met with soon after and she was phenomenal. She also made me feel comfortable and acknowledged that while I was very young, it was extraordinary that I was taking my future seriously and into my own hands. She expressed to me that while many other surgeons would be apprehensive and a bit more conservative due to my age that was not her place to make these choices for me. It was her job to give me the best chance at life possible. I had my team and I was very excited to move forward. In making this choice, I considered that I wanted to live a full life, to have a career that I love, to have a family, and to not let cancer interrupt any of that. While I knew that I could not possibly control every other possible interference, I knew that I could substantially reduce my risk of this one thing.

I knew that I wanted to have the surgery while I was out of school for the summer so I had to schedule it accordingly. Before my surgery could be scheduled I had to have a breast MRI performed to make sure that I did not have cancer already. I had the MRI done and it took about a week to receive the results. The emotions that I felt during that weeklong waiting period helped to solidify my choice. I could not imagine having breast scans and appointments every six months and waiting for results twice a year. Personally, that is not something that I could handle and I knew that I needed to go through with this surgery to be at peace. I received my MRI results a week later and my scans were normal.

On to scheduling...

This was the most difficult part of the process because they had to coordinate both of the surgeons' schedules and mine. My surgery was eventually scheduled for July 25, 2012. That would leave 3 weeks to recover before school began for the fall semester. I spent my summer enjoying my family and my boyfriend and doing things that I thought I would not do for a while after my surgery. I went to the beach often, I played miniature golf, among many other things.

July 25, 2012.

I arrived at the hospital at 5:30am to check in for my surgery. During the days leading up to my surgery I had not been nervous. On the morning of, the nerves finally came. I remember sitting in the admitting office tapping my feet and wringing my hands. Okay, I was not nervous I was terrified. Here I was, 23 years old, with my natural breasts that I loved, they were healthy, and I was having them removed. I felt crazy. I went into a room where they put a wristband on me and the woman who checked me in just so happened to be a family friend of my boyfriend. She gave me just what I needed. She calmed me down, she put me at ease, and I felt confident in my choice again.

Shortly after I was whisked away to pre-op where I changed, had my IV inserted and answered thousands of questions. After about an hour they let my family come back one at a time to see me. My dad came back first. We joked around for a minute as we always do. I wanted to cry but I knew that if I did he would cry too, so I held it in. He hugged and kissed me and then my mom came back. My mom, being the tough woman that she is, was just who I needed to see in that moment. I finally cried. I was not crying because I was scared to lose my breasts, I cried because I had never had major surgery before and I am sure that the fears that I had were completely normal. She put everything into perspective and made me feel much better. Finally, Alessandro, my boyfriend, came back to spend time with me. He stayed with me in pre-op for the remainder of the time that I was back there. My breast surgeon stopped by and said good morning and then my plastic surgeon came back and began to draw on my breasts where the incisions would be made. It was not until this moment that I realized this was really happening. Alessandro and

I spent the remaining minutes laughing and trying to make light of the situation. The nurse came over and gave me a "margarita". I began laughing hysterically as they wheeled me back. I remember being in the operating room and getting on the table. I remember meeting the nurses and after that, no memories remain.

Unfortunately, my surgery did not go as planned. It had been decided that there was no need to do a sentinel lymph node biopsy since my breast MRI was normal. I had a fear of lymph node removal seeing the nerve damage and pain that it had caused my mom. However, when my breast surgeon was performing the mastectomy on my left breast, she noticed something troubling. The lymph nodes in my left arm were black. She dissected eight lymph nodes and feared that I had melanoma. She and my plastic surgeon later told me that it really scared them and they could not believe what they had seen. Fortunately, it turned out that I did not have melanoma and that ironically, the lymph nodes in my arm had soaked up pigment from my breast cancer ribbon tattoo. Other than that, the mastectomy was complete and the expanders were put into place with a little bit of fluid inside of them.

The first thing that I can recall after waking up is my breast surgeon telling me about my lymph nodes. I remember being upset but I did not fully digest the information until later. I just wanted to go home. They gave me some more pain medication, I put my clothes on, and I was headed home just a few hours after I had gotten out of surgery.

I got home, got right into my bed and felt so relieved. It was over. The pain was not too bad and my chest looked noticeably smaller but I am sure the pain medication helped me cope. I never felt much pain throughout my recovery. But I was not free of complaints and frustrations. The worst pain that I felt came from the drain tubes. I had two drain tubes and they dug into my ribs because the surgical bra was so tight. So, when I would sit up, I would pull the bra away from my skin to give myself a little bit of relief. Another frustrating part of my recovery was that I was unable to sit up on my own. I would need to get up but I could not muster the strength and I would need someone to lift me up. I was very determined to recover fast though. After about three days I started to slowly wean myself off of the pain medications and I walked often. We live in a very quiet and secluded residential neighborhood where everybody knows each other. I would go outside, in my pajamas, and walk up and down the street. I had never experienced such a radical procedure, so getting back to my active self took time and that was quite frustrating, but I was determined. I had some visitors, a lot of messages and phone calls and all of these helped me heal quickly. I felt so much love and support and it really made the healing process more manageable.

After eight days I had my drains removed and Alessandro took me on a date to celebrate. Having the drains removed involved minimal discomfort. I only felt the removal of the stitches holding them in and after that it just felt weird as they were being pulled out. I was free! I now understand why most women told me that the drains were the worst part of the surgery. This was also the first time that I saw my chest in all of its flat glory. I went from a C to an A and it was very different, but it felt kind of nice. I was most excited because now, without the drains, I could finally take my first shower. It took me about five days to really be able to touch my chest. It was almost painful but mostly uncomfortable at first but I have since gotten used to it.

Three weeks after my surgery, I began my second year of law school. I am writing this today, 12 weeks after my surgery and half way through my semester at school. I have already had my expanders filled three times. I am getting bigger and starting to look relatively normal in clothes. The expanders are mostly uncomfortable, as they are rock hard and oddly shaped. The expansions are quick and they do not hurt during, but I do experience some pain and soreness in the first few days after. I have a long way to go but I am just so relieved that the hardest part is over. I have been able to get back to running, playing tennis, and have no restrictions at this point. At the end of 2012, once I have finished final exams, I will have my exchange surgery where I will have my rock hard expanders removed and have them replaced with nice, soft, silicone implants in addition to fat grafting. After I heal I will have nipple reconstruction with tattooing and my journey will hopefully be complete. I am extremely anxious to see the final result. I know that they will look amazing and I am extremely confident in my plastic surgeon's abilities.

My journey in becoming a previvor has taught me so much about myself as well as about others. I have learned that not everything goes as planned. I also learned a lot about patience. I am always seeking instant gratification and this, being a process, has taught me to be patient. People often asked how I could remain so positive throughout this and how I was able to continue on with school and what they did not realize is that being negative and quitting was never an option for me. To me, this was just another thing that I had to get through. I know that once I get through it all I will be a stronger person. The way that others supported me throughout this process has touched my heart. My parents, my boyfriend, my family, and my boyfriend's family showed me unconditional love and did anything they could to help me. Lastly, but definitely not least... The Pink Moon Lovelies. I have never met a group of strangers who had so much love for one another. This selfless group of women is there for one another no matter what time of the day, to give advice on any matter and to comfort one another. Many friendships have resulted from this group and I really do not know what I would have done without their love, support, and advice in addition to my friends and family. I decided to be very open about my journey, although very personal, in the hopes that I will be able to raise awareness and help others. I know that my choice was a radical one and that it is certainly not right for everyone.

I would like to conclude my story by thanking my parents, Rhonda and Robert Surber, for taking time away from their jobs to take care of me and for catering to my every need including driving me to appointments. I also want to thank Alessandro for being by my side and helping me through this by supporting me every step of the way and reminding me that I am beautiful no matter what. Thank you to my friends and family for the outpouring of love and support and to my doctors and nurses who have provided me with exceptional care and guidance. And a special thank you to Nicki Boscia Durlester. Thank you for sharing your story and creating a safe haven for women, using social media, to discuss their innermost feelings, their fears, their concerns, and creating a place for other men and women touched by cancer to share their story. You are an angel on earth.

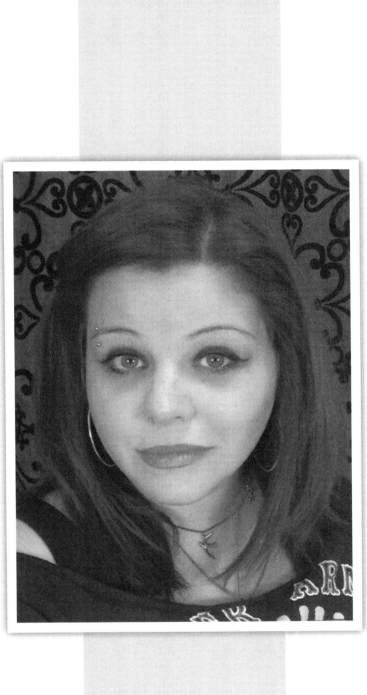

Rachel Harrison

BRCA1 Previvor, 31
Chaska, Minnesota USA

Work In Progress

Memories of being a little girl usually include dressing up in your mommy's clothes, bracelets, necklaces, earrings and high heels. For me there was one more memory, dressing up in mommy's fake breasts. Some of my oldest memories are of my mom struggling with cancer. I don't recall all of the specifics, but within the first six months of my life my mother received the devastating news that she had Stage IV breast cancer. She was 29 years old. They believed she had developed breast cancer in 1981 when she was pregnant with me.

Mom was recommended to have surgery and chemotherapy. She was told that Stage IV is an advanced cancer and although she should fight she needed to be realistic about her prognosis. According to the American Cancer Society, women who have advanced breast cancer at the time of diagnosis live approximately 18 months after diagnosis (median survival rate). In 1981 that survival rate was even less.

Having just giving birth months earlier with two other young children at home, mom was not about to become a cancer death statistic. While raising her three children with my loving father, mom went through surgery to remove her cancerous breast and lymph nodes followed by chemo. Shortly after mom's diagnosis my maternal Aunt Jan was diagnosed with cancer as well. Thankfully Aunt Jan survived and went on to raise a beautiful family. 1983 brought great news. Mom had beaten Stage IV cancer. With the cancer threat gone our family life proceeded as normal until 1994 when my mother was diagnosed with cancer in her other breast. They found it earlier then the cancer in 1981. After going through chemo mom once again beat breast cancer.

In the summer of 2000 Mom began experiencing abdominal pain. After a few doctor's appointments and thinking she had a nasty flu she was diagnosed with ovarian cancer. She went through surgery to have the tumor removed and a complete hysterectomy. Due to her history of breast cancer mom decided to have genetic testing done to determine if she had hereditary cancer. She tested positive for the BRCA1 mutation. Her oncologist talked to us about the recurrence rate of cancer when you have the gene and urged our family to have the BRCA testing done. I remember feeling so overwhelmed with the information I was given. My sister seemed to accept the information with such grace and courage. I on the other hand felt like I had been hit by a bag of bricks. From the minute I found out about the genetic mutation I had a sick feeling in my stomach that I had it, as if I had always known. The feelings went back to those days of wearing Mom's breasts and thinking it was perfectly normal, always believing cancer was a normal part of a woman's life.

While Mom was going through chemo we found out that my maternal cousin Karine had been diagnosed with breast cancer. She was 26. Like Mom, Karine also tested positive for the BRCA1 mutation. Karine and my mother both went through chemotherapy. After a year of treatments Mom's cancer went into remission until a few days into the New Year of 2003 when her health took a rapid decline. Upon a visit to the emergency room it was discovered that Mom's ovarian cancer had returned and this time it was terminal. After a month in hospice my mother lost her battle to cancer at the age of 51 and I lost my beloved mom and best friend. Three years and one day after Mom passed away cousin Karine lost her battle with cancer at the age of 34.

The pain that cancer brought our family left us all feeling like we needed to be smarter about our health. That is easier said then done. The journeys of Mom and Karine left us with more information on how to screen for cancer and be aware that it can happen at any age. My Aunt Jeannie started yearly screenings including the blood test for ovarian cancer known as the CA125. My mom had encouraged her to do this so her doctors would have a baseline to go by just in case.

In the summer of 2008 I began following the story of Amy Taylor, a young woman who had been diagnosed with breast cancer when she was pregnant with her child. Amy was making videotapes of advice, stories and conversations for her kids just in case she didn't make it. She knew it was important. She even bought gifts in advance, drew pictures and other special things for them to have. When I started following Amy's story I had three young girls. Her fight and desire to always be there in some way for her kids left me feeling that I needed to do what I could to be here for mine. I needed to get the genetic testing done. I needed to know because knowledge is power. If I had the gene I could do things to help me live a long life with my family. Shortly after making this decision I found out that my other maternal aunt had been diagnosed with fallopian tube cancer. This was a wake-up call for our entire family. As if losing Mom and Karine hadn't been enough we were not about to lose Aunt Jeannie.

I had the BRCA test and after what felt like the longest three weeks of my life I found out I had the BRCA1 genetic mutation. Aunt Jeanine went through her surgery and did testing as well and found out she too had the BRCA1 mutation. After testing positive I immediately wanted to do what I could to be here for my family. While waiting for my surgery date my other maternal Aunt Joanne had a mammogram and was diagnosed with early stage breast cancer. She was also positive for the BRCA1 mutation. She decided to have both breasts removed with reconstruction. Fortunately, she did not need chemo.

In late 2008 I had initial meetings with my plastic surgeon and breast surgeon to discuss the options of reconstruction surgery. There are so many options and far too often the serious risks are glossed over. I was not told of any potential complications that could arise from the surgery I chose to have. I had my prophylactic double mastectomy and reconstructive TRAM flap surgery on February 25, 2009. My breast surgeon removed my healthy breasts and my plastic surgeon used stomach muscle, tissue, fat and skin to reconstruct my breasts. The surgery was over ten hours long. There were issues with my blood vessels connecting to the new tissue. Failure of the vessels to connect would result in necrosis of the tissue. If the blood vessels failed to connect they would stop the TRAM surgery, close me up and wait to consult with me about implants. After several attempts my surgeon successfully connected my vessels and completed the surgery.

I was released from the hospital a week after my surgery. The day after I returned home I was in really bad shape. I had never been sicker in my life. I ran a fever that spiked up and down from 97 to 104 degrees. I went to the emergency room where I was admitted to the hospital and given antibiotics and fluids. The next day my surgeon operated again to take a look at what was going on. He found a massive infection that was rapidly spreading. The doctor was concerned with the proximity of the infection to my heart and how aggressive it was. They cultured the infection, which turned out to be a MRSA staph infection. They did their best to clean up the infection and instead of sewing me back up, they put a wound vacuum in so they would be able to revisit and maintain the infected area. I spent the next week with a 4" x 8" gaping hole in my abdomen while being administered intense antibiotics. I had five more surgeries in an attempt to clean up the infection. I was in the hospital for a month before asking to be released to be home for my daughter's 10th birthday. I was sent home with PICC line in my arm for antibiotic infusions. I was on antibiotics for two and half weeks, 12 hours a day with a visiting nurse every two days.

It was a lot to go through, but having the surgery significantly reduced my risk of developing breast and ovarian cancer. I wish someone had told me that complications could happen. You watch fictional TV shows and see things like this without realizing it can happen to you. Due to the slow healing from the infection and the additional surgeries my scars and body did not heal the way it should have. The first few days after my initial surgery I was thrilled with the results of my reconstruction. I was, however, left with very large raised scars and a disproportional stomach. My stomach muscles are very weak and often look like they are bulging out of my abdomen.

Since my surgery in February 2009 both of my aunts had reconstruction surgery and complete hysterectomies. All of my mom's siblings have tested for the genetic mutation. We found out that all six siblings have the BRCA1 mutation. My Aunt Jeannie's cancer went into remission. Out of 16 cousins in my family six cousins have tested for the BRCA1 mutation. Four of us are positive including my cousin Karine who passed away.

On January 5, 2011 I had a complete hysterectomy. It was one more step in the direction of doing everything I can to be cancer free. This was such a difficult choice to make, even harder than my breasts. This would take away my ability to have more children and put me into full-blown menopause at 30 years old. Hormone replacement is an option but there are conflicting studies whether BRCA positives can safely take them to minimize effects of menopause. While having my hysterectomy my plastic surgeon tried to fix the bulging muscle in my stomach. He corrected it but my stomach still doesn't look great.

I am thankful I reduced my risk of breast and ovarian cancer, but it has not been an easy journey. My surgeries had a big impact on my self-esteem. A big issue with woman my age is how to address this with new partners. Some of us have chosen to abruptly end our childbearing years. How do we have normal love lives when we don't have the sex drives we had prior to surgery? What date do you bring this up on? Do you ruin the spontaneity of seeing each other for the first time by telling your date what to expect? There are people who view preventative surgeries as mutilating. It is hard for some to understand that our breasts and ovaries are like ticking time bombs. I for one would not keep a bomb strapped to me waiting for it to detonate if I knew it could be removed.

As of November 2012 I am still a work in progress and plan to have revision surgeries to fix my bulging stomach and improve the look of my breasts and abdomen. It will probably be a few years before I am done with the procedures and able to move forward with my life. The unfortunate thing about this genetic mutation is that even with preventative surgeries there is still a slight risk of getting breast and ovarian cancer. I am not free of sleepless nights and worry. Recently I found a suspicious lump. After a clinical breast exam and MRI it was determined to be fat necrosis and scar tissue. The necrosis is painful and I hope to have it removed as soon as possible. I also have lymphedemea in my arms. Lymphedema is a condition of localized fluid retention and tissue swelling caused by a compromised lymphatic system. Tissues with lymphedema are at risk of infection and it often causes a tight painful feeling in the affected area.

I know I have a journey ahead, but I remain hopeful for a cancer free life. It is my hope to give back some of the love and support I have received from all of this. I hope to encourage the rest of my relatives to test for our mutation, as it is aggressive in our family. There are options to reduce the risk of hereditary cancer and there are many great support groups for guidance. I encourage anyone with a family history of breast and ovarian cancer to seek genetic counseling and find out the right steps for you.

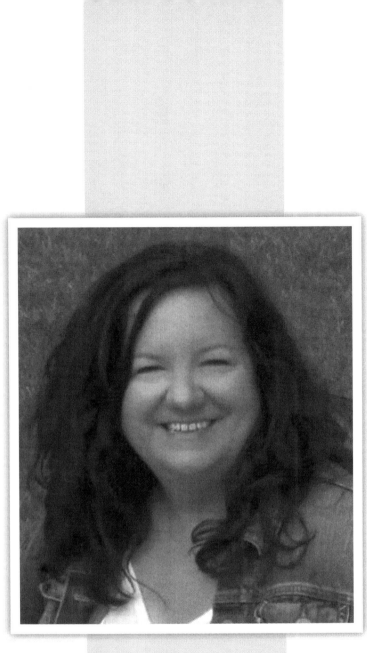

Sara Bartosiewicz-Hamilton

BRCA2 Previvor, 35
Kalamazoo, Michigan USA

Five Years

I grew up fearing the Big C (for the record, we called it that before there was a show). My mother's side of the family was riddled with cancer: breast, ovarian, lung, pancreatic, and colon. I never knew my Nona (Italian for grandmother). She died of breast and ovarian cancer before I was born. Even to this day, my mom and her siblings will tear up when they talk about watching helplessly as their mother passed away from this terrible disease.

When I was a teenager, I was brought to the hospital to see one of my aunts. I was told this would probably be the last time I would see her. Miraculously my aunt is alive and well today. She was the first one in the family to be tested for the BRCA mutation and was positive for BRCA2. My mom tested positive shortly after her, which meant I had a 50/50 chance of inheriting the mutation as well.

At that point in my life, I was dealing with secondary infertility. I had given birth to our son, but had been told shortly after that I shouldn't expect to become pregnant again because of a hormone disorder. I knew I could not deal with both the secondary infertility and the gene mutation so I set it aside.

Several years went by and we were blessed with our second miracle baby. The realization I was approaching my 30th birthday woke me up. I knew the earliest age of onset of cancer in the family was important. I had a cousin who found a tumor at 30. I knew it was time to be tested.

I received my positive gene mutation results in the fall of 2006. On January 18, 2007 I walked into the pre-surgical room terrified if I would come out, terrified of what I would be if I did come back out.

January 2012 was my five-year "anniversary" of my prophylactic bilateral mastectomy. Here is what I wrote:

Here I am...

I am terrible at keeping track of time and dates. This month continues to shock me as I watch it fly by. I had in the back of my mind that today was fast approaching, however, when I looked at my phone this morning, I realized TODAY is THE day!!

On one of the message boards, someone referred to their anniversary as a "boob"iversary. Well, that is better than anything I can come up with and it made me laugh when I read it. I love to laugh.

Five years! It is amazing to me that it has been that long, and there is a part of my brain that finds it hard to believe it has only been five years. A lot has changed since that moment.

The morning of my surgery, I woke up holding my breasts. I think subconsciously I was saying goodbye. I had never held much stock in my breasts. I was an A cup until children and then, well, they were "I've breastfed two kids" C cups, but it was the appreciation of knowing I fed my two children, bonded with them. I was thankful for the opportunity.

Waiting in pre-op was pure torment, emotionally and mentally. The nurses and doctors kept asking if I wanted anything to help calm down. Naively, I kept telling them I would be fine. When they came to get me I lost it. I just started sobbing as they wheeled me down the hall. I was so terrified. It was the unknown. Not knowing what to expect, not knowing how I would feel, not knowing how I would look. Anticipating the pain is always worse for me than the actual pain. And now a part of me looks back and thinks I must have been sobbing for feeling as though I had no choice. The choice I made felt like the only good choice I had and it wasn't feeling like that great of a choice.

It took me a week after surgery to gather enough courage to look. I was lucky my family came and took care of me. My hubby made it his mission to do whatever he could to help alleviate the pain both physically and emotionally. I spent the week letting him deal with the dressings and the drains (disgusting!) and I would simply turn my head so I didn't have to look. He kept asking and I finally told him I was ready. I wasn't, but I think we both knew I could not continue ignoring my new reality. As I sit here trying to type this I'm crying as I remember the girl who was terrified at what she saw. I sobbed, wailed and remember looking in the mirror and being so upset at what I was. I felt as if I had lost me. I went and heaved trying to get control again, trying to forget that it was my body I had just looked at.

The next few months I was pretty out of touch with the world. I physically hid away in my home. Mentally and emotionally the pain meds helped me escape. I was going through the expansion process and it hurt like hell, but honestly I know there was part of me just not ready to face what this was and what it meant.

I know I have said it before, but it is worth repeating, to someone who never gave a thought to her breasts prior to her prophylactic bilateral mastectomy (PBM). It became annoying as the next couple years were consumed by constant doctor visits to reconstruct what was no longer there, to make sure that what is left isn't going to develop into cancer. I think it annoyed me because I never got the chance to forget. It is amazing how good I have become at having a mental "black box" to hide my memories of my breasts. I don't see them. I have to consciously tell myself to look, but the constant appointments with everyone lining up to see never let me forget. I chose not to see but they were still there.

And that is what my life was, maybe still is, an attempt to be proactive and at the same time shove my head in the sand. I did what had to be done and hoped the rest would go away and take care of itself. It didn't at least for me. It didn't....

I have always hated when someone tells me to write a letter to myself five years from now, ten years from now, as if the me in this moment has ANY idea what or where I'll be years from now. These questions bug the crap out of me because I'm a "bad" adult. I don't do well making decisions based on a long-term future. I do better being spontaneous and quite frankly I am becoming more comfortable with the thought that I may never know what I want to be when I grow up. I just plug along and believe I'll be exactly where I'm meant to be. Well today I am thinking I hate these questions because I look back and I can tell you, five years ago I would have NEVER had ANY idea who I would become from the moment after my PBM.

I have always been a writer. So as I began my journey I turned to writing as an outlet. I didn't have people around me who were ready to deal with what was going to be my reality and I didn't have the strength to train them in time to be supportive. So I started writing and I thought if I am dealing with this someone else is probably dealing with this too. I began posting my blog and letting an intimate piece of who I am and where I am out into the world. I quickly learned there are people who will try to use this against me and I had to make a choice. Do I let them send me running back into my house shutting myself away, or do I give them the virtual finger and keep on? I think you realize what I chose. I chose to make my journey about more than my breasts. I will never be okay with the thought that I had to choose to have a PBM to make my odds against the Big C better nor will I allow myself to curl up into a fetal position and let it be all there is.... end of story. I decided I had to do for me whatever I could to help the girls and women who would walk a similar path after me. Trying to help others became a better reason for my journey. It gave me a sense of purpose and helped me start to make peace with it all.

I started working with Bright Pink, founded around the same time as my PBM. Its mission is to help educate and support women with my gene mutation. When I found Bright Pink I felt as though I found my "club". The organization is EXACTLY what I had needed when I was facing my surgery. I needed to be connected with a young woman who had gone through a PBM and I began to volunteer to be that support person for other women. Women who are questioning whether or not they want to go through genetic testing and women who have found out they are positive and questioning what to do next. I wanted to support these women as they make the choices that are right for them.

I posed for the SCAR project. At that moment, I had to step away from the keyboard and bare it all. My intention for posing was for women going through the same process I had. It was so frustrating for me to not find any photos of a young woman who had a mastectomy. I was terrified going into surgery because I truly had no idea what I would come out looking like. I had taken photos of myself at every stage so I would have them available should someone ask to see, but I wanted to participate in a project that would reach women on a much bigger scale. I went with the intention of showing women who are facing a PBM that, yes, you will look different than before but you will be okay. I went to New York City for those women. I was scared and nervous. What would my parents think? What would my children think? What will all the conservatives I grew up with think? What is my husband going to think? But, in the moments before my photo, I began to think, oh my God, I am about to take off my clothes in front of these strangers. My sister is about to see my scars. What is SHE going to think? What is HE going to think? What are THEY going to think? They are going to see my scars. I am about to show them my scars!! I am not really sure I breathed. I remember David Jay, the photographer, telling me to stop blinking (it's a family thing) and to loosen my face. I was trying not to cry and kept telling myself to breathe. I survived. I showed my scars and no one ran away screaming. In fact, they opened their arms and welcomed me, supported me, and showed me my scars would not define our friendship or me. I went to New York City to help other women. I came home from New York City changed.

This has been my journey. With every telling of my story, I get stronger. With every criticism my resolve grows deeper. Five years. Five years of sitting with other women, crying with them, supporting them as they face their journey. Emailing and letting women know they are strong enough to make the choices they feel they should. Standing in a gallery with the portraits of my SCAR sisters, sharing my story, showing my scars, signing my portrait in the book, five years of writing my blog baring a piece of my soul that doesn't see daylight in my "real world".

Five years. It was five years ago when the most difficult decision I ever made became my reality. I cry because it was traumatic. The actual surgery, the reconstruction, and the direct ramifications of not having my own breasts, cutting off a piece of my body, have been incredibly difficult on many levels. Five years of facing the fact there are people in the world who say they are your friends but aren't really. Five years of meeting some of the most kick-ass women and then watching them leave the world. I cry because I will never know another day where all of these things are not in my reality.

Five years. I cry because I am so incredibly overwhelmed by the beauty in all of this in spite of the trauma. Five years of realizing what life is and isn't about. Five years of being able to explore whom I am and what defines me. Five years of meeting some of the most kick-ass women and David Jay. Five years of knowing there are people who "get" it. Five years of feeling unconditional love, support, and acceptance. Five years of finally being on a path of self-acceptance.

I would never have imagined on that day, January 18th, 2007, that in five years I would have the peace and love of who I am and where I am. My life is not perfect, far from it. I have lots of lessons I need to learn but seem to be hung up on ones I can't seem to fully grasp. But I am okay. I survived. I can wholeheartedly say I would not trade these past five years for another five years of my life before. It wasn't easy but is anything worth having easy to get to? I am not going to limit the possibilities by hypothesizing what may be in another five. Instead I'm going to sit back and reflect, be thankful, cry these tears and say...here I am.

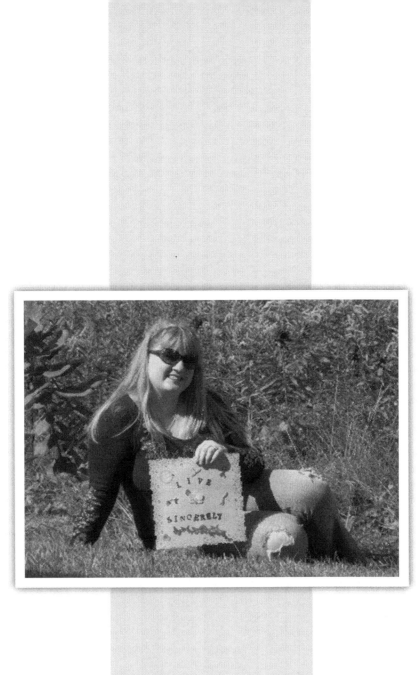

Helen Smith

BRCA1 Previvor, 41
Ohio USA

Where Dark Meets Light

For as long as I can remember, cancer has been a part of my life. At the tender age of three, I can remember sitting on a tricycle outside watching the medics taking my grandma away on a gurney. My next memory of her was in the hospital. They allowed me to see her even though I was so very young. She gave me a glazed doughnut that day. It was the last time I would see her alive.

Throughout my life I have lost many people to cancer, including loved ones, friends and neighbors. It wreaked havoc all around me. My mother, Velma, found a lump in her breast at the age of 35. It was malignant. She had a lumpectomy and was watched closely for a while after she had chemotherapy and radiation treatments. I was attending Northern Kentucky University at the time working on an art degree. I decided to put my college education on hold so I could work and be there for her.

Her next occurrence was not long after that. I think she was 40 when it showed up in the other breast. This one was different.

It seemed more aggressive, as it was in her lymph nodes. She had more treatments and her lymph nodes removed, and again with surveillance afterward. She was a trooper, fought hard through the second battle and lost her hair again. Her faith was strong and we thought she beat it once again. She had little issues in between and was never a complete picture of health, but seemed to be doing okay. I must say, looking back, I wondered why she never opted for mastectomy, but now that I'm an adult I realize that she watched her mother go through a double mastectomy in the late 60s/early 70s, only to suffer a horrible death at the hands of metastatic breast cancer.

April Fool's Day 1996, she had been complaining of headaches. Her arm would also jerk wildly and involuntarily. Her doctor called it a pinched nerve when she saw him in previous visits. That particular day the headaches were unbearable, so she went to the hospital. They did a brain scan and found she had metastasized brain cancer. The oncology doctors said it probably spread after her first occurrence. Both of my aunts and I were literally floored. I sometimes think I was so caught up in the stress of it all that I really didn't know what to do to help her. Thankfully my Aunt Meg was there every single step of the way, going to appointments, searching out new doctors and possible treatments.

After we got the news, the battle was on! She tried chemo, radiation, shark cartilage, and many other types of treatments. My stepdad and I, aunts, in-laws and many of her friends stood by her through this difficult time. In the last year of her life she lost use of one side of her body. In the last months of her life she had to have 24-hour care. We took shifts and had a hospice nurse there to help so she could stay home as long as possible. During that time, my mother and I made peace with each other for things we had done in the past to hurt one another. I remember the day they took her to the hospital to stay in the hospice unit. It was a Saturday. She wasn't eating and could barely speak. That day was the last time she verbally told me she loved me. I went to the hospital every day to see her, as did my aunts and stepdad. The doctor would come in daily and say he'd be surprised if she made it another day. I felt so angry with him for saying those things in front of her. She would show him up by being alive the next day. After a couple of weeks of watching and waiting, she would only go when it was time, her time. I used to curl up on the bed around her feet and brought in my best teddy bear. He was a giant white bear with big cheeks, so Mom called him Cheeks. Mind you, I was 28 years old and felt like a child! The day mom passed, I had gone to see some friends to try and take a little break from the hospital. She waited until my Aunt Meg and I weren't in the room and she passed away with her friend Ida and my Auntie Pat there with her. I remember the phone call, but don't remember how I got from where my friends were to my mother-in-law's home. I fell into my sister-in-law's arms sobbing uncontrollably. This awful monster had taken another precious life in my family... my mother.

One year later I left my husband and relocated from Kentucky to Columbus, Ohio. Since then I have had my yearly mammograms and female exams as recommended. In 2001, I heard of a genetic test that you could take to see if you have a predisposition to breast cancer. With my family history I sort of knew what the results would be, but really wanted to check it out. The test was too expensive at the time so I held off. At the age of 35 I found a lump in one of my breasts and about lost it. I was dating the man who is now my husband. He can attest to how distraught I was. Was I now doomed to the same fate as my mother? As it turns out, it was only a fibrocyst and went away before the oncology doctor saw me.

Years later, the BRCA test came back into my life through my Aunt Meg. She found a group of women who had also been dealing with similar issues. Cancer has always been part of her life too. She and I began researching it once again. In 2008 we decided to meet with a genetic counselor, along with my Aunt Pat and my husband Terry to discuss our family history and our options for testing and what comes after. We went through the counseling but none of us acted on it at first. A year later, my Aunt Meg went to a conference in Florida through a group called FORCE (Facing Our Risk of Cancer Empowered). When she came home, she convinced me that I really needed to take the BRCA test. It was logical in my mind that I should be the first for many reasons, and then if I tested positive it would pave the way for the rest of my family to test. In May of 2009 I tested and got my results in July, BRCA1 positive. Even though I knew in my heart I was positive, it didn't stop me from breaking down right there in the office. I remember leaving the office, calling Aunt Meg and telling her the news. We cried a good bit over the phone, and she thanked me for going first.

The confirmation was life changing to say the least. I came home that day and told my husband. He looked at me and said, "Babe, it's a no brainer, you have got to have the surgeries." I had already begun researching the different types of mastectomies and toyed with the thought of surgical menopause long before the test. I felt like I had to be prepared ahead of time so whatever the result, I was ready to make an educated decision on the matter. I was actually okay with the hysterectomy part; no more menstrual cycles would be a welcome thing. Also, I knew there were hormone patches to help with the side effects. I also made a point to get my mother's medical records so I could learn more about her cancer. She was triple negative, which is the most difficult form of breast cancer to treat. I cried my way through reading her medical records; which is one of the hardest things I've ever had to do.

At the time all this was going on, I was taking a biochemistry course for my degree, which was quite helpful in learning the science behind the diagnosis. I did a good job of putting BRCA in a nice clean little clinical box. I went on FORCE's website and found the "Breast Reconstruction Guide" by Kathy Steligo. What a blessing! I had a source to help me ask the right questions and educate me on which procedure I wanted. I decided on the DIEP (Deep Inferior Epigastric Perforator Flap), which meant I was going to use my tummy to reconstruct my new breast mounds. My thought process was if I'm going to go through all this I might as well get some aesthetic benefit (flat tummy)! I was also more comfortable with the DIEP because my breasts would still be my tissue, a part of me if you will. I had a prophylactic salpingo oophorectomy and hysterectomy over Labor Day weekend. Getting rid of my uterus and cervix was not an issue for me, as a uterus is used to carry a child, which at this point wasn't ever going to happen for me. There was no sense in risking cervical cancer. The surgery was laparoscopic, meaning the doctors only had to make small incisions to remove everything, and the recovery would be short. I went back to work in six days. Once I set my mind on something, I feel it's best to get it done and move forward. I also scheduled my breast surgery right away. This allowed us to take advantage of meeting our out of pocket expenses for the year for our insurance, and it was a good time to be away from work.

I thought choosing a doctor would be a no-brainer. Once I decided to proceed, I made appointments with the same institution that did my genetic counseling. I liked the oncologist, but didn't really know the plastic surgeon, except that he had good credentials. The oncologist was scheduled out until November, but I was willing to wait. Upon seeing my plastic surgeon, I met with one of his associates. I had already done my homework and knew exactly what I wanted to do and had my list of questions. The lady was shocked and jokingly said, "Well there goes my speech." She did give me some helpful information that wasn't already on my list. She proceeded to tell me about the team of people who would be in charge of my care, and the numerous appointments I would have once I decided to move forward. She was very kind, but I couldn't help but feel rather slighted that I wasn't meeting with the surgeon, even if for just a brief moment to introduce him to me. This procedure was at a minimum 10 hours long, so I felt if he was going to operate on me, especially such a delicate and long procedure as the DIEP, I wanted to, at the very least, meet that person up front. After all, it is my life that would be in his hands.

After that visit, I decided to get a second opinion. I googled "Doctors who performed DIEP procedure" in my city and found Dr. Wong Moon on 'Locate a Doc'. I put in a request to meet with him. He called me that same day without even having an appointment first. He was very informative, as was his staff. They were forthcoming with a reference; I didn't even have to ask. He took great care in speaking to both my husband and I about complications, how many procedures he had done, what can go wrong, and what has gone wrong under his watch. Needless to say, my husband and I were both very pleased to have found him.

The plastic surgeons work with particular doctors depending on the hospital network they are in. This also addresses the oncological side of things, since being BRCA positive makes you a high cancer risk. His nurse set an appointment for me to see Dr. Alicia Terando. She was very informative, caring, and knowledgeable. She recommended a nipple sparing procedure. She assured me that the tissue would be scraped so thin that the breast tissue of the nipples would be gone, nearly eliminating most of the cancer risk associated with the nipple. What was left was just a skin representation of my former nipples. We also discussed taking a few of my lymph nodes to make sure I didn't already have any nasty little cancer cells hiding in them. If things looked suspect, she would go for the sentinel nodes, but if not, she wouldn't risk my having lymphedema to take them. It turns out she only had to remove one node, which was great news for me.

Immediately after the hysterectomy I was using a .050 Vivelle Patch. I was a train wreck without hormones. By train wreck, I mean hot flashes galore and weepy, sad, moody ALL of the time. The littlest things would send me into a crying spell. My libido was also pretty much gone. So I had to plead my case somewhat for hormone therapy. I was relieved (as one could imagine) when my doctors agreed it was okay, since my breasts were going to be removed anyway. After my breast surgery, I started noticing around February or March of 2012 that I was having those weepy-for-no-reason kinds of spells and called my OBGYN. I asked her to increase my hormones, as I think that was my problem. Mind you, when life happens, I can usually take it in stride when my body is in balance. This wasn't the case. My doctor agreed to increase my hormones, and since then I feel much better. It simply amazes me what estrogen can do!

December 7, 2009 rolled around, and it was time for the DIEP. My Aunt Meg and Aunt Pat were there with my husband Terry through the entire ordeal. They spent the night before my surgery with me. We stayed up until 2 or 3 a.m. talking about all sorts of stuff. We laughed and cried through the night. My Aunt Meg brought me a care basket of things I might need post-surgery, along with a prayer shawl made with love by her friends. I had that shawl with me through the entire ordeal. I still have it safely tucked away. I was nervous, but happy to have my loved ones there with me. I was told that I was out for 17 hours, as my right nipple wasn't being cooperative and almost died. Due to my touch and go nipple, I was in ICU for 3 days.

When I got to my regular room and was by myself for a little bit, I had to take a peek. It was a surreal experience, but it wasn't so bad. I thought I'd feel rather odd about my breasts, but they didn't look too bad. I sort of chuckled when I looked at my tiny little flat belly. I was also pleasantly surprised that Dr. Moon was able to give me a belly button. The staff all took great care of me during my stay; they even brought me a heated shower cap that you put on your head to sort of wash your hair, since I couldn't shower. It's funny how we take every day things for granted like clean hair. I sort of felt like a science experiment for a little bit, as I had so many doctors, nurses and interns coming to see my new breasts. Modesty goes out the window after such an operation.

During my recovery, my husband Terry was such an amazing force in my life (he always has been). He handled all of this so well. He brought me my meals, showered me and helped me get dressed. He put up with so much, but asked nothing in return. We had purchased a recliner specifically for helping with my recovery from this procedure. I slept in the recliner for three months. I hated it, but at the same time was so thankful to have it. The anesthesia took several weeks to wear off also. For the first month I couldn't do much but watch TV. I was unable to focus long enough to read books or do any other activities from my chair. The only time I would get out was for doctor appointments. I talked on the phone with friends and some visited me. I also discovered the BRCA Sisterhood during this time, as I had nothing else to do while in recovery. What a wonderful group of ladies! I am forever grateful to them for inviting me into the fold. I got so much great information from FORCE, but then went to the sisterhood and got so much love by women who knew exactly what I was going through.

The next phase of the journey was the stage two portion of my breast surgery. I had little patches of skin that looked like eyes on my breasts they are called skin flaps. It's where the doctor can keep an eye on the skin to make sure it isn't dying. I was fortunate that the only complication I had was my wonky nipple. In May 2010, I had my stage two surgery where the doctor closed my skin flaps. There would only be a single line scar on the side of my breasts. Liposuction would smooth out my sides and little poochy areas in my tummy and groin. After some roadblocks that could not be helped, I made it through stage two and was on my way to the all done club. It's interesting to note through this entire journey I was still attending classes and working on my Bachelor of Science degree. My point in saying this is if you want to achieve something you can, no matter the life circumstances.

I do not regret my decision to be tested or to have these life altering/saving surgeries. BRCA is a large part of my life, but I no longer sit in fear waiting for the proverbial boot to drop. There is still an amount of aftercare one should consider after having these surgeries, such as bone density checks, vitamin D levels and cardiovascular health. I learned a great deal of this through the many BRCA related groups; most notably the Beyond the Pink Moon Facebook group, I belong to. I truly believe God blessed this part of my life and will use it for good. I give lectures to students about BRCA and try to advocate when life allows it. What seemed like a curse was also a great blessing. It is an honor to have forged so many relationships with some of the most amazing women I know from all over the world. Had it not been for BRCA, these would have been lost opportunities, so for that I am thankful!

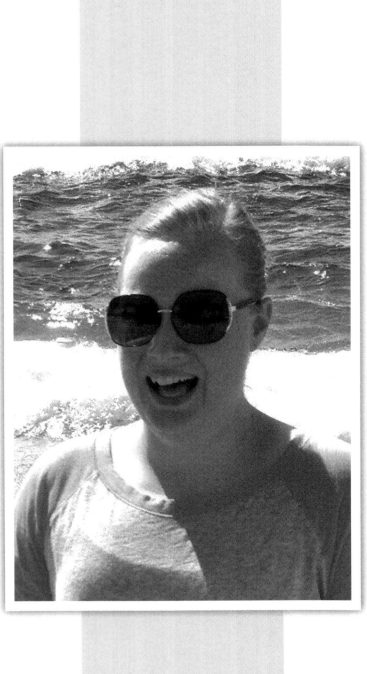

Heather Grinde

BRCA2 Previvor, 26
Seattle, Washington USA

Quarter Life Crisis

When I was eight years old I took a stab at writing in a diary. If 90s sitcoms had taught me anything, it was that all girls have diaries they kept under lock and key between the box spring and mattress. You know, that clever hiding spot that no one else would ever think to look. I remember sitting down and cracking open the little pink stiff book. The pages were lined and waiting for me to fill them up with my inner most thoughts.

The number 2 pencil dwarfed my young hand and the weight of that added Lisa Frank eraser almost made it impossible to hold upright. Nonetheless I pressed the graphite to the blank page and wrote about my day:

Dear Diary (*capitalized of course, because it is her name after all*),

Today was a sad day. My great grandmother died. Also, I was jump roping and a small piece of dirt flew up and got into my eye. My eye was really red and hurt a lot. Today is a bad day.

Love,
Heather

I know what you're thinking; I was obviously a gifted 2nd grader! Alright, getting back to the story, aside from my early intellect. I closed Diary that day and placed it under my mattress. The next day I knew I was supposed to open Diary up and write again. Instead I used the little key to open her and re-read what I had written the previous day. I started laughing and thought how silly this concept really was. I considered that I would be so embarrassed to have someone else read this. That was the last time I ever wrote in Diary.

I couldn't wrap my mind around the whole concept of writing down daily recaps and feelings of the happenings of my little life, especially if I was just going to re-read it and be embarrassed of myself.

It took a long while before I began to understand the therapeutic healing of writing. However, I still do not keep a diary or journal privately. I guess I feel my words are best used when read by others. That may sound like I think I have something so important to say and that it is my civic duty to enlighten you, but that's not at all where I'm going with this.

You see, I'm convinced that each and every one of us have invaluable life experiences and lessons we can share with one another. I really do believe that old sentiment that even if you just reach one person, you'll have made a difference. Sure, that's the teacher in me, and maybe you disagree, but if anything, my written words are helping me, so I've already won.

It is with that build up that I share what's been going on in my life recently.

"Dear Heather, you had single site BRCA testing and you tested positive for the 1417ins4 BRCA 2 mutation. Positive for a deleterious mutation."

Uh, what? English please. As I continued to read down my test results letter I began to slowly understand the weight of that statement.

"Being a carrier of a BRCA2 mutation means that you have up to an 85% lifetime chance of breast cancer and a 27% chance of ovarian cancer by age 70."

When I received this letter, it had been two weeks and two days from the day I had my blood drawn to be sent to the lab, in order to be tested for this mutation. For those of you who don't know, BRCA stands for **br**east **ca**ncer. The mutation I tested positive for is often referred to as the breast cancer gene (mutation). I was referred to a genetic counselor because my mother tested positive for the mutation a few years ago, which meant I had a 50/50 chance of inheriting the deleterious mutation. I guess the glass was half empty in my case.

I received my initial results by phone from my genetic counselor a few days prior to receiving that letter. The entire two weeks after I had my blood drawn and sent for testing, I knew that it was going to be positive. Not because I'm a pessimist, but because I just knew. I can't explain it much more than that.

So now comes the hard part. What do you do with information like that at 24 years old? I have at worst, a 15% chance of not having breast cancer by 70. What? In addition, BRCA mutation carriers have an elevated risk of ovarian cancer too! Which by the way is one of the deadliest and hardest to detect cancers, period. Not to mention, the cancer that took my grandmother's life. She also carried this mutation passing it down to my mother, and her to me.

The months that followed the news of my positive result letter were filled with research. I became consumed with information about anything and everything BRCA related. I read books, I scrolled message boards, I frequented chat rooms, and even met other BRCA carriers locally. It only took me about a year to decide that a bilateral prophylactic mastectomy is what I needed to do.

I was terrified that my friends and family would react adversely when I shared with them my thought process behind why I needed to have a mastectomy. However when I began telling my story, I was met with empathy, understanding, and love. You see the reason it took me only a year to decide to have surgery is because I had had eight surgeries prior. I knew what it felt like to be chronically ill and the thought of an impending cancer sometime in my life was more than I wanted to bear. I also understood how much of a mental toll this knowledge was taking on me. I was only in my mid-twenties, yet I was thinking about breast cancer multiple times a day. In the end, quality of life was the deciding factor that sent me to the operating room.

At the ripe age of 26, I was wheeled off for my prophylactic bilateral mastectomy. I wasn't scared. I didn't cry. I knew that I would be fine. I woke up after 7 hours of surgery and felt the pain. That pain was quickly diminished by all the adrenaline and pure euphoria I felt when I realized what I had done. I had taken a preemptive strike against breast cancer. I had cut my risk down to single digit percentages. I had removed the gray cloud that had hung over me for the past year and a half. I had pre-vived breast cancer.

My BRCA journey is not over. I will live with this for the rest of my life. As I get older and finish having my family, I will visit an OR once again to have my ovaries removed in hopes of diminishing that cancer risk as well.

The road hasn't been easy, but that's life. I've experienced more in my short 26 years to date than most of my peers, and that's fine by me. I was given an opportunity that earlier generations did not have and with that, I chose to live. To live fully without the weight of fear holding me back. How fortunate am I?

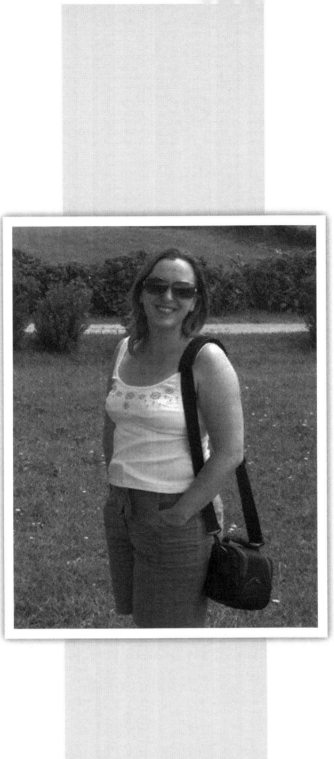

Jackie Coleman

BRCA1 Previvor, 32
Surrey, UNITED KINGDOM

Facing Up To Reality

2007

The day started much like any other working day, although I remember feeling quite pleased with myself for getting in early for once. The phones were already ringing and the office was buzzing. I was idly checking through emails when over the phone system came an announcement, in a very jovial voice, from one of the guys covering reception. "Jackie you have a phone call." I laughed as I picked up the phone. The line was quiet. Then my mum spoke. She could hardly get the words out. She had found a lump in her breast and had made an urgent appointment with her general practitioner (GP) that day. "Don't worry" I tried to calm her down, "Let's see what the doctor says."

Later that day when I called her she informed me that the GP was sending her to the hospital for a biopsy later that week. Okay, I thought. If it was serious surely they would biopsy straightaway. Nothing to worry about.

At the end of the week when by sheer luck I had beaten the traffic and got in early again, I was surprised that the idiot covering reception was joking around saying I had a call on the line. This time I could hear uncontrollable sobbing. I don't know how my mum had managed to speak to the goon on reception, but it must have been all she could manage. Between sobs I heard the words, "I have breast cancer." I told her that I would call her back after I had sorted some things out at work. I put down the phone, my heart was in my throat, and calmly walked towards my manger's office. It was empty. Fat chance he would ever get in early. I walked on past and spotted the director sitting behind his desk. I knocked and walked in. Before I could even say I really need to leave work to take care of some family emergency, which I had been rehearsing in my head, I just burst in to tears. He handled it brilliantly. I now found myself sitting in his chair with a box of tissues. How embarrassing. Pull yourself together. But I couldn't get the words out. Between sobs and sputtered words "mum" "breast cancer" he understood. Next thing I know, the goon from reception appeared. He would drive me up to my parents. They weren't going to have me driving in the state I was in.

I managed to compose myself by the time I reached my parents house. I somehow managed to talk my mum through how we would cope with chemo and getting through the next few months. After my mum had her tumor removed a sample was sent for genetic testing. Women from my mother's side of the family had not fared well in the battle against breast and ovarian cancer. My mum's test came back positive for BRCA1 mutation. This wasn't a surprise.

2008

My mum finished her last round of radiotherapy two weeks before I got married. On my wedding day she looked amazing and tried to hide her fatigue and exhaustion. After I came back from my honeymoon she handed me a letter from her genetic consultant. The letter advised getting a referral from my GP to my local genetics clinic for BRCA testing. I didn't live locally to my mum so I couldn't go to the clinic where she had been tested. I took the letter and put it away in a drawer. My mum kept asking if I'd had the test for weeks afterwards. I always had the same answer "Don't worry, I'm on top of it." It wasn't that I was being lazy; I just wasn't sure what the testing would mean to me. The more I thought about it the more anxious I got.

Soon this anxiety began to manifest in other aspects of my life. I became nervous in public. I couldn't make decisions. I eventually went to my GP and explained it all. She prescribed Prozac to overcome the depression and anxiety. It was what I needed to get out of the door and ask for the genetics referral. I stayed on Prozac for the next year and after a few counseling sessions and anxiety management stopped taking it.

2010

I'd asked for a genetics referral at the end of 2008. I was sent a letter inviting me to attend a consultation in January 2009. I cancelled. This happened three more times. Eventually they said to call when I was ready. I waited until the summer of 2010 to finally pluck up the courage. My sister had taken her test a few years ago when mum had given us the letter. For the past year and a half I'd had my sister and husband begging me to go and have the test. My sister had been diagnosed as BRCA positive. She was only 26 at the time and would have to wait another 4 years for screening. She tried to convince me it was no different than cervical screening. It's not the same. Women in our family get breast cancer. Fact. I knew my result would be positive. Call it a self-fulfilling prophecy. Waiting in the outpatient's clinic I knew the result. I spotted the genetics counselor coming out of the room. She met my eyes and I knew. When she called us through I just blurted out" Well it's positive isn't it?" "Yes" she confirmed. I felt her and my husband's eyes boring in to me. They were waiting for a reaction. She handed me a box of tissues. I just placed them on the desk. "It's okay to cry," she said. I didn't feel like crying. And that was the start of taking control. I wasn't going to be a quivering wreck. I did have a few private moments, but I tried to think this through logically. The only option was for surgery.

2011

I spent most of 2011 in consultations with the breast surgeon over a mastectomy and my reconstruction options. Well most of the appointments were about the reconstruction. I was having the mastectomy. Just how my new boobs would be made, well that was the hardest decision. I had to use every ounce of courage and determination to kick back my anxiety and resist the urge to either crawl into a deep depression or do something far worse.

I did want a DIEP reconstruction. Unfortunately I didn't have enough belly to make reasonable sized boobs. Great. Actually a blessing in disguise. Implants turned out to be the better option for me and would mean that my abdominal muscles would be fine if I decided to have children later down the line.

In September 2011 I had my surgery. All the anxiety disappeared with the breast tissue. It's been a journey like a rough patch at sea. I've weathered the storm and am now safely coasting in to the harbor. I still have to think about having the expander implants exchanged and nipples! I never considered having a tattoo and now I'm thinking about 3D nipple tattoos!!

I've never tried to talk my sister into having surgery. I just try to talk positively about my experience with the surgical team and how I feel about breast cancer now that I've had the procedure. I want her to make her own choice. Inside I'm screaming for her to have the same. But it's her decision. I can only show her how it could be.

2012

My exchange surgery date couldn't come soon enough. Expanders are unpleasant and uncomfortable. I had my exchange to silicone implants in February 2012, surprisingly as day surgery. It felt amazing. I awoke from surgery, chatting to the nurses in recovery and asking for a cup of tea. I made it on to the ward just in time for lunch and after polishing off a sandwich and some fruitcake they let me go home. Recovery was swift in comparison to the mastectomy. The relief that came following the exchange surgery was unbelievable. My breasts felt soft. I couldn't stop prodding them. I did have two very large, red scars though. I began applying vitamin E oil in earnest, anything to make them fade or disappear. A week after the surgery I was back at work. I felt like a new woman, with a renewed feel for life and a deep appreciation for my health and living a life true to my heart's desire.

A few months after the exchange I went back to the hospital to talk about nipple tattoos. It felt like the right time. The nurse did an amazing job, matching the colors and deciding on the size. I trusted her judgment on these factors. I had no idea how large my nipples should be or what was the right color. I will need a bit of a color touch up soon, but I'm leaving it a few months. I don't like feeling like a slave to hospital clinics. There's no rush.

A year since my mastectomy and I don't regret my decision. I still feel empowered. I feel strong and more confident about my body than I did before. I've made strong connections with others who have traveled the same path, bonds that will never be broken.

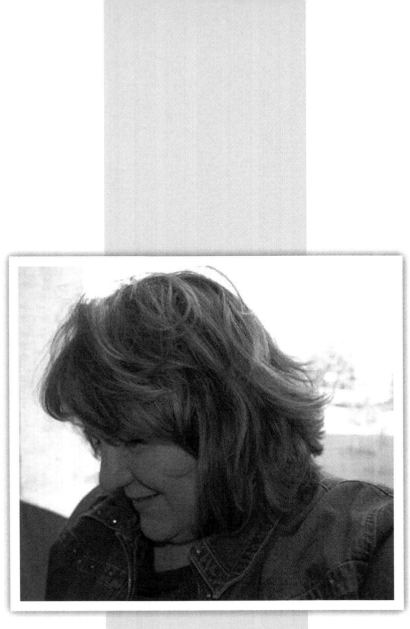

Patricia Peters Martin

BRCA1 Previvor, 53
Quantico, Virginia USA

I'm A Mutant

I have to start at the beginning to make sense of the end. My father is from Kansas and had been in the United States Navy for ten years when he met my mother. She was a North Carolina Southern belle who was on active duty in Great Lakes, Illinois. They fell in love much to the chagrin of my mother's family who wanted her to wed a Southern boy one day. When they married and she became pregnant with me she had to get out of the military. Women could not be active duty and pregnant at that time. She was a young 20-year-old mother away from home. We were stationed in Hawaii when she had my brother. He was premature. His placenta was embedded in her uterus so she had to have a hysterectomy, though they left her ovaries. Since she was only 24 she had to take hormone replacement therapy (HRT).

I only visited my mother's family a few times since we were a military family and moved around. I never knew her father. My mother's parents divorced when my mom was young, at a time when that rarely happened. She was close to his family members and

I do remember them. We settled in Kansas while my father was in Vietnam and stayed there after his retirement from the Navy.

Growing up I never heard the word cancer unless it was in hushed tones and never of the breast. When I was fifteen my mother had been painting the house and told me she had found a lump on her left breast the size of a golf ball. I was a bit taken aback as she had never talked about body parts with me. The idea of anything being wrong with her was truly foreign.

She consulted with doctors at Fort Leavenworth who decided to operate. They were certain it was breast cancer. She had her left breast removed. I can remember sitting in the waiting room and not much else. The next day when I went to see her she was walking down the hall laughing and saying she was ready to come home. Amazing! She started chemotherapy and it made her very sick. When she started to lose her hair she cried a little. She never cried again in front of me. She thought it was great fun to answer the door with her bald head when someone would come to visit, just to see their reaction. We had assumed she had developed cancer at 36 due to the hormone replacement therapy. Once the chemo ended she went on with her life and graduated from college with a degree in History and Education. Her dream was to teach high school history.

When I was twenty I joined the Navy. Around that time my mother found out she had ovarian cancer. She was told they were baffled at why she had two primary cancers. She was written about in the medical journals at that time. Due to Fort Leavenworth being a small military hospital she had to be medevacked to Denver to Fitzsimons Army Hospital for more surgeries and treatment. My mother made this trip several times. Often I would take leave and stay with her in Denver. She was amazing. She would walk around to all the patient's rooms each day to visit and check on them. I would go with her on her rounds when I was there. It was so fun to see her laughing and joking. She knew everyone's story and cared for all of them. I still never thought she would die. I had not lost anyone close to me and she was so strong and so positive all the time. We would make our time together an adventure by talking, reading, doing needlepoint (hard for her to do with lymphedema) and ogling the military men in the chow hall. She was a riot! I stayed with her through treatments and even when they had to drain fluid from her lungs. Regretfully whenever she brought up the topic of her death I would always change the subject and tell her nothing was going to happen. Foolish me...

I was stationed in California and had orders to go to Hawaii. I was pretty excited about that. One day my detailer called me. He was my former Commanding Officer and knew of my mom's illness. He said he could send me to Great Lakes so I could be close to my mother. I did not have to think twice. I already had my orders and port of call to Hawaii but being nearer to my Mom was the choice for me. I was due to transfer in August around my 23rd birthday. I had talked to my mom the second week of July. She was so excited I was coming home and would be nearby. She had many birthday plans for me. A week later the Red Cross call came that my mother was dying. They flew me on the red eye out of San Francisco to Kansas City. I made it to the hospital 30 minutes before she died. I was with her. It was so hard. My brother, also in the military, made it to her room 15 minutes after she passed. My world turned upside down. I knew she had cancer but never in a million years thought she would die. For many years I would reach for the phone to call her and realize I could not. It took many years for me to be able to even say the word cancer. Did I learn anything? Was I doing my own breast exams? No.

A couple years later my maternal grandmother died of a sudden stroke. I was a married, with two young children and lost contact with my mom's sisters after my grandmother's death. There had always been a bit of distance in our families but the connection was lost for a long while until 2010.

My brother John and I are very close. We had talked about our mother's family a lot and it seemed they were on our minds more the older we got. He found my cousin Ashton on Facebook! She is the daughter of my mom's middle sister. She accepted both of our friend requests and proceeded to tell us that her mother and their younger sister had battled breast cancer two and three times. They had been tested for the BRCA gene mutation in 2003 and were found to be positive.

The mutation was traced to my grandfather's side of the family. It was 2010; I was 50 years old and just finding out about this. I was horrified and glad at the same time. This is why I lost my mother. I also could have been struck down at anytime. I was able to reconnect a bit with my aunts. I was tested in July 2010 and was also positive for the BRCA1 mutation. Thankfully my brother is negative. I had my ovaries removed in November 2010 and both breasts removed in February 2011. The reconstruction failed. I developed septic infections on both sides and one side ruptured. Although the expanders were removed and I was disfigured, I would still do it again. The relief of not suffering and having my family suffer cancer was and is tremendous.

In June 2011 I went to my first FORCE conference. I met so many wonderful women. It was amazing. The life changing part for me was the night of "show and tell". Inside a private area women volunteer to show their surgical results. I saw the whole gamut including implants, DIEP and women who chose not to reconstruct. I was impressed by all. I had been leaning a bit toward having scar revision and getting rid of the excess skin and staying flat as the infection had left me sick for a long time. I got my affirmation that night. Each and every one of the women was beautiful and comfortable in their own skin. But here is the life changing part... there was a young women who was photographing women for other BRCA projects. She had an area closed off and women were going in taking their tops off and getting photographed. I thought maybe it would be good for others to see what happens when the surgery is not quite right. Up to that point I hated looking in the mirror when I was nude from the waist up. It made me cry. I was glad to be alive and never have to worry, but I was horribly disfigured at that point. So I held my head up and went behind the curtains. I was met by bright lights and the face of a lovely young woman with nothing but compassion in her eyes. I took my top off, stared into the lights and let her take the pictures. Then she said, "Now look... you are beautiful." I looked at her and then looked at the camera and I was bowled over. I did look beautiful, strong and determined. I broke down. I will never forget the compassion in the photographer's face. I wish I remembered her name. Through her photography I came to a place of healing. I am forever grateful.

A month later my daughter was tested. She is also positive. She is very strong and informed. At this time she is choosing active surveillance. There is no hurry for her since she is aware and has the knowledge.

I thank God each day we were given this information. I have met so many wonderful people and it has been so good to share this connection. It is a double-edged sword. Good to have the information yet very scary to think of the ramifications of it all. I am trying to forgive my aunts for not trying to find my brother and I. It is tough. Although they are not very involved in our lives, we try to keep in touch with them. I have regrets about not listening to my mother and not accepting I could lose her. I do not regret my surgeries and the ability to save the lives of my children and their children. I now am involved in breast cancer and ovarian cancer organizations along with FORCE. Finding out I have the gene mutation has been a gift. A gift of life and of healing. I had my revision surgery December 2011 and love how I look! Now I nag all the women I know to check their breasts each month. I thank God each day for all I have.

Jessica Bremer

BRCA2 Previvor
West Monroe, Louisiana USA

Moving Forward

My story begins long before I was born. It began with what was thought to be the family curse. I will explain that "curse" through those that made me.

My personal breast cancer story begins in the late 1960's when my grandmother, Mary Jo, was first diagnosed with breast cancer. She was a single mother of three children. She underwent a mastectomy and chemo. It didn't take long before they realized that she couldn't take chemotherapy because it burned her veins all the way through. So immediately during her first chemo session, it was stopped. She was a fighter though. The cancer seemed to be contained and she survived 16 more years cancer free.

In 1984, while my mom, the youngest child and only daughter in her family, was pregnant with me, my grandmother found out her cancer had returned. It was in her bones, and incurable. My grandmother, never the one to rock the boat too much, didn't want to interrupt her children's lives and chose to tell no one. I think she was worried what this news would do to my mom, who was pregnant with me at the time.

Right after giving birth to me, my mom found out she was pregnant again. I was only four months old! My grandmother stayed quiet. She came to our house on a Tuesday when my little sister was two weeks old. She took my Mom outside and told her she was going to the hospital and wouldn't be coming out. Her cancer was back and this was the end. Yes, she kept it a secret from the family and her friends for two years. Two weeks later she passed away. She lived just long enough to see all of her grandchildren born. She was 54 years old.

That is the curse. No woman in my family had ever lived past 54 years old. Breast cancer seemed to always get you first. It is a known in our family that you will live a good life, but at 54 or before you will die of breast cancer. I was very young and remember none of this, but it is has affected me because, I am so much like her. I still to this day, 25 years later, get stopped by ladies in the grocery store asking if I am related to her. I look just like her. I am told we even have the same mannerisms and quirks. In knowing this I have always assumed I would be the same. Live a good life and die at 54 of breast cancer.

Fast forward to 2008, I had just gotten married the year before and was expecting my first child when my mom found the lump. And guess what she did? She told no one!! I had Mary Kensli in April and my older sister got married in June, and the week after my Dad came to my house. It is about 30 minutes from my parents, so I thought something was up. But I had a two month old, so visits are often and unexpected. He hung out for a little bit then said, "Jessica, I have to tell you something. Your mom found a lump in her left breast and is having a biopsy done tomorrow." I had never before had a moment in life where my world just stood still, but I experienced it then. I froze, my heart froze, and my world froze.

I knew immediately it was cancer. So the next day, I went to the hospital and waited for the biopsy. After, the doctor let us go in as he personally carried Mom's biopsy to the lab. About 10 minutes later, he returned. He walked in and said, "I'm sorry. It's cancer". There my world goes again. I cry, my daddy cries, and my mom says, "Can I get dressed now?' REALLY? She was so calm and collected. I now know it is because she understood. You see, my mom was 54. She was turning 55 in October. She had already accepted that this was it. She only had a few months left. And knowing that nothing made me madder! Dang curse!

Mom had a mastectomy the next week and started chemo soon after. Chemo was so hard. She had six rounds and it almost killed her. Her second round of chemo sent her into multi-organ failure. She ended up on a ventilator in ICU. At this point, they didn't know if she would come out of it. I had a 12-week-old baby, my husband had been activated with the National Guard five hours away, and my sisters were both living out of state. I was alone. I was all alone in this world.

I had to go into that hospital room, while a nurse outside held my newborn (my mom worked at the hospital so I wasn't a stranger) and tell my Mom goodbye. I had to tell her that it was okay if she left me alone in the world. Truth was, it wasn't okay. I was a newlywed, with a newborn, I had just graduated college and I needed my Mom. I needed her here. I walked into that room, and I wouldn't tell her it was okay. Everyone told me to tell her, but I couldn't. As I walked out of that room and picked my baby back up, I remember feeling so alone. It was that moment when I began to hate cancer. It is not that I ever liked it, but it was a part of our lives. At that moment, I realized that in just a few short years, that could be my daughter and me. At that point I hated to even hear the word Cancer.

My mom came through it, and went on to do four more rounds of chemo. They all made her sick. She was in multi organ failure three more times and on life support two more times. Each time they gave us bleak chances. Each time she fought through. These months are all a blur to me. I can't remember most of it. I think the stress was too much. We had moved in with my parents to help take care of my Mom. I hate that I don't remember this, because I don't have any memories of my baby being a baby. But I do remember my mom turning 55! Yes!! The curse was broken and I was so glad it was my Mom who did it!!

In June of 2010, I went to get my yearly checkup. My nurse practitioner (NP) is a friend of my family and our moms have been friends for over 30 years. She knew the whole family history and she asked if I had ever been tested for the BRCA gene. I had never really heard about it. I had heard there was a gene after my Mom was diagnosed, but her oncologist made it sound unreliable and probably a waste of money. He was my grandma's oncologist and my Mom's. Jessica told me it was reliable and referred me to have the test. I told her if it was positive, I would have a double mastectomy immediately.

I scheduled my appointment and my husband and I drove to Shreveport, LA (one and a half hours away). I talked to the genetic counselor who went through the history. I left after having my blood drawn. The next week I received a letter in the mail explaining that according to my family history and the chart, along with my age and good health, I have an 8.7% chance of having the BRCA gene. I breathe a big sigh of relief! That's a 92.7% chance that I don't! That is an A in school!!! There is no way!

We went back the next week to get the results, which I "knew" were negative, however she told me I am positive for the BRCA2 mutation. My mind froze. "What? Positive? What about 8.7%? There is no way!" I kept thinking that, but nothing came out of my mouth. I couldn't speak. I had never been speechless in my life! She spoke to me about a doctor for a prophylactic bilateral mastectomy (PBM) and I stopped. I didn't want to remove my breasts. I was 25 years old. I had a two year old!

When it became real, my plans weren't as clear-cut as I thought. I really struggle with this whole BRCA thing. I began getting tested and on my first MRI, I got called back for an ultrasound. Then another ultrasound. Turned out nothing, but I got scared.

I haven't tested in almost two years now. I am afraid of what they might find. I am also not ready to give up my breasts. I hate them and I know they will kill me, but they are MINE. God gave them to me! They are small and ugly but they are MINE.

My mom was diagnosed with metastatic breast cancer of the bone last year and is now Stage IV. My step grandmother (who has been the only grandmother I have had) passed away from complications from her metastatic breast cancer three weeks ago. See even if you marry into this family it gets you!

My husband is ready for me to have the PBM, although he believes it is ultimately my decision. He does not, however, want to have this hanging over our heads indefinitely. He does not want to be a single dad to Kensli. As fate would have it he won't be. I recently found out I am pregnant again! I have another appointment with my oncologist because it is required by my OB/GYN. Our second child is due in May 2013. My husband will deploy in August 2013. When he returns home from his deployment we will plan for my PBM. Although I feel more ready now, I don't think I will ever come to terms with this lousy gene, but I will move forward. I will push forward! BRCA2 will not define my future or me.

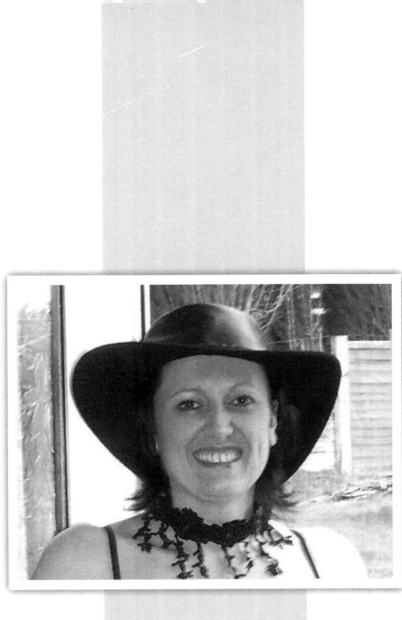

Amanda Johnson-Birks

BRCA2 Previvor, 42
Cornwall, UNITED KINGDOM

Green Light Flashes

My BRCA journey began from a medical point of view at 3:35 a.m. on January 28, 2002. From that day onwards my entire being has been overshadowed by love, losses and the fear of breast cancer all relating to C.859+2T.G The gift that just keeps on giving!

Let's rewind a little first though, without going into too much detail, looking back my childhood was always a little obscure in comparison to other children in my neighborhood. I suspect their families spent weekends at the park, cycling or baking with Grandma. My childhood was spent hiding behind doors and listening to whispered conversations of my Mum on the telephone to one of her sisters. A family of eleven, five sisters and four brothers, Grandma and Granddad and an extended close family of great aunts, uncles, and second cousins twice removed yadda yadda.

Anyway nothing unusual about that, you may think, except one of the first words I ever managed to find of my own accord in the dictionary was cancer. Why? Because it was a name, a phrase and soon to become a report or in my own world a watchword or a secret code that told me "not for children's ears."

Green light flashes. Do you wish to take on this mission? Okay then what is cancer? Any dreams I had of becoming part of the Secret Seven or Famous Five were soon to be dashed. At 11 years old I fully understood inside and out what it meant to have cancer. For as long as I could remember my grandmother was always in and out of Hospital with various gynecological problems. Not long after I watched my wonderful grandma deteriorate before my eyes. In a short space of time she was admitted to the hospital and the cancer that had been residing in her body for most of my childhood had indeed taken its parting shot by finally grasping what was left, thus leaving my whole family devoid of our lovely grandma. She was 58 and to this day I will always remember the smell of lifelessness.

Within ten years, my great aunt then passed of breast cancer at 50. Another great aunt died of ovarian cancer at 52. My Aunt T, who was more like a sister to me than any other, passed of liver cancer at 32. I was alone with her when she died and I thank her for that. Following this my second cousin then passed of breast cancer at 32. Not to mention my great grandmother (another casualty of breast cancer) at 50.

This is where I can only reiterate that an awful lot of my adolescence was spent around my cursed family. I seem to recall my mum's family were then given a short respite and for the first time ever I seem to remember some kind of normalcy taking hold, and although we were all grieving in our way, we were still able to function as a family and try with all our might to become "normal," whatever the hell that was.

I look back now and can fully understand the meaning of Damocles Sword. As a family we had been living beneath it for as long as I can remember. However, that "sword" came crashing down with such force on the morning of June 8, 1997 when my wonderful mother came and told be she had found a lump in her left breast. Okay, I told myself, let's keep it together. My mum after all was feigning extreme courage and assured me that she wasn't worried and nor should I be. She had already made her doctor's appointment for the following morning and all would be well.

The day before her doctor's visit she and I spent the day outdoors and the unwritten rule of that day was NOT to mention it. It was NOT going to spoil our day. How naïve I was. I actually believed all would be well and that following our family's recent history, it was not medically possible for another cancer diagnosis. Wrong again! Long story short, my mother underwent a biopsy. Results = malignant growth. Solution: due to the size of this growth the removal of this breast was necessary including all lymph nodes. Operation successful! Mum returned home with a supply of Tamoxifen to be taken every day for five years. Oh and a very obscure looking fake breast for her bra. Boy did we share some laughs over that!

Time frames I'm not great with these days, but I do know within the space of a year my mum had made her decision to have reconstructive surgery on her left breast and even that surgery proved successful and after a long recovery, I recall being able to breathe a long sigh of relief and tell myself it was over. My mum had won that battle hands down and I secretly wanted no more than to stick my middle finger up at cancer there and then and send it on its way. We had after all accommodated this disease for long enough and by then it had out stayed its welcome by far.

For four years my mum and I became absolute best friends. We did everything together and even though we lived only a few doors apart, when we were not together we were continually on the phone laughing and making plans for the following day. Gradually though, things began to change. Slowly at first, in fact so slow that life carried on as always except for the fact that Mum was becoming extremely breathless and couldn't walk very far. Another doctor's appointment resulting in a diagnosis of asthma and came home with an inhaler! Short walks down the garden, were to no avail, nor even a shower without a shower stool.

Asthma my ass!

A further visit to a doctor for a second opinion suggested that whatever the problem was further investigation was needed. As Mum was still under the care of her oncologist, a return visit was scheduled. Routine tests were carried out, including all kinds of x-rays, mammograms and MRI scans. Return of the oncologist poker faced, lacking any kind of compassion reads almost from a text that the cancer had returned and had now taken residence in the lining of my mum's lungs! Yes Mrs. B, we will start you on a very aggressive course of chemo, but feel at this time your cancer has probably progressed to Stage IV. God if I could have five minutes alone with that female oncologist, even today I would be tempted to kick her ass into next week! Mum was as noble and brave as ever. I was falling apart inside and started to binge drink in secret, realizing what a total coward I was. I hated myself, kept my abusive marriage a secret and prayed as hard as I could for God to take me and spare my mum. Chemo started, my mum shaved off her own lovely hair, not allowing the chemo to take it from her. I grew to understand the patterns and what to expect every three weeks, regarding sickness and fatigue and good days before beginning the whole cycle again.

Chemo ended and as I recall, it was just a waiting game from that day on.

From here on in though, our waiting game didn't actually play out for that long as Mum then started complaining of extreme back ache and loss of breath again. Her lungs were filling up rapidly and oxygen was needed everywhere she went. Hospital appointments became a regular occurrence. By this time she was having her lungs drained twice a day. This offered little comfort as by then my mum's health was already on a downward spiral.

A short visit home was much looked forward to, and bed really was all the medicine needed. News travels fast within a hospital environment and by this time mum already knew that her secondary cancer had in fact taken its second parting shot on the generation map and would soon be taking with it my wonderful mum. During this time, although in extreme pain and fighting for every breath, my Mum planned her own funeral, wrote final letters to her loved ones and made me promise to mend bridges with my estranged father, so she wouldn't be leaving me an orphan. Her battle with cancer ended June 6, 2002 at 6:06 a.m. in a hospital room full of family members. She was 53 years young.

I won't bore you with the details of what happened in my own life afterwards. It really isn't great reading material and by then I was in a very bad place anyway. I will continue by fast-forwarding a little bit to the year of 2004. Someone in the medical profession picked up my family history and had some kind of a Eureka moment as things started to move frantically from there on out. Phone calls were made from one department to the other, which was fast-tracked even more after one of my mum's remaining sisters was diagnosed with uterine cancer at 56. Thankfully she made a full recovery and has since tested negative for the gene.

I was invited to have one of those informal chats where gene mutations were explained fully to me. Many of my mum's remaining family had the same chronicles explained to them, followed by only a few of us undergoing the genetic testing offered. Another remaining sister of my mum tested positive. My Aunt E followed this up by having a full Hysterectomy and prophylactic bilateral mastectomy (PBM) in March 2005.

One of my mum's brothers also tested positive for the gene and is currently waiting for his children (my cousins) to have the test. Another brother tested negative leaving two other brothers and another sister that have chosen NOT to have the test. It would seem that to date they would rather not know their fate.

Incidentally, the faulty gene WAS found in my mum's blood sample, which brings me to my own positive BRCA2 result. The Golden Egg! My brother has chosen not to have the test. He would rather not know.

Hand on heart and for reasons I cannot explain nor fathom I already knew prior to entering the consultant's office that my result would be positive. My aunt who accompanied me that day almost fainted when she heard the result. She was the one in need of medical attention and ironically not myself. Maybe this is why she has since opted out of genetic testing. Unfortunately like many families our own family crumbled at the seams after my mum passed and many of us are no longer in contact with each other. I have no further information to offer. I have since found out though that my younger first cousin, who I believe is four years younger than me, was diagnosed with breast cancer last year at 35 and has since had a double mastectomy. I am unsure whether she was actually tested for the gene, although I know her father, my uncle, tested negative. End result I was 25 and struggling to hold down an abusive marriage and offer a normal life for my three children, who were transforming into teenagers over night. I didn't have time for surgeries and allowed myself to believe that I wouldn't have the support anyway. I opted for strict surveillance against the advice of my medical team, having the CA125 test every three months, mammograms every year without fail, and cervical screening. You name it, and I had it with bells on!

I participated in the United Kingdom Familial Ovarian Cancer Screening Study. I agreed to donate samples of my own blood for storage of biological material and possibly for us in further research. This involved a blood kit being sent to my home address every three months, and having to take it to my GP for him to take blood before I had to package up three blood filled tubes to dispatch at a strict time, allowing it to arrive at another disciplined time at the research university it was to be held. Strict health questionnaires also had to be filled in methodically during these times. Time management worked well though. I found myself on an even keel and eventually trained myself to switch off from blood tests, and although still struggling with grief I did actually pick myself up and stopped myself from dwelling on breast cancer and my own mortality. My children grew up quickly and I found the courage to leave my marriage, packed as much as I could in the back of my car and literally re-invented myself hundreds of miles away in a new area, new county, new job and new friends. Even now I have no regrets of choosing surveillance when I did. Thankfully in all of that time I didn't ever encounter any serious abnormalities. As I turned the big 40 the worries I believed were laid dormant reared their ugly heads and I began to think more seriously about possible consequences especially as my child-rearing days were coming to a head.

That still silent voice in my head was becoming louder every day. I began to worry that perhaps I had tempted fate for too long. Now that I was in a loving relationship with Steve did I really want to take the chance of having breast or ovarian cancer when I had been given the chance to reduce my risks and defy the odds of a long and painful illness? I also have to state at this point due to my own personal belief as the years progressed I began to realize that it wouldn't be a case of IF but rather WHEN.

August 23, 2009 was the day I had both ovaries removed via keyhole surgery. No regrets there apart from the fact that I was thrown into surgical menopause overnight. Hot flashes became overwhelming and my chin resembled a not so miniature Schnauzer, but a small investment into a damn good pair of tweezers sorted that little problem. HRT, weight gain, multiple stomachs and a feeling of continuous bloating often makes one feel a little despondent, but I am a work in progress and I am trying so very hard to overcome this problem. Small price to pay though in the grand scheme of things don't ya think? So I'm not sweating the petty things here.

In February 2011 I finally stepped through those hospital doors and had my PBM! I must admit my real breasts and I didn't have a great relationship to start with. We never actually bonded. They were never "money makers" but more spaniels' ears. I actually had three nipples, so I guess I'm quite fortunate as possibly a few hundred years ago I might have been burned at the stake for this.

Anyway my surgery went well, as did my immediate reconstruction with saline implants. My fills were hilarious and even now remind me of a bicycle pump. I have the occasional down day, as I'm sure we all do. I still find myself becoming angry or upset at not having my mum around, and having to make these awful decisions without her, but then I'm reminded that she didn't have these choices. She wasn't given the option of choosing life, I was!

I can look at my children and hopefully one day my grandchildren and tell them that I did everything I could to prolong my life. I can remind them that knowledge really is power and that one day a cure WILL be found, but until then trust in yourself, listen to that small still voice and do whatever you have to do to keep the fear away from your door.

Life is precious. Embrace it with everything you have and more. Remind yourself that life is not measured by the amount of breaths you take but by what you put into those breaths.

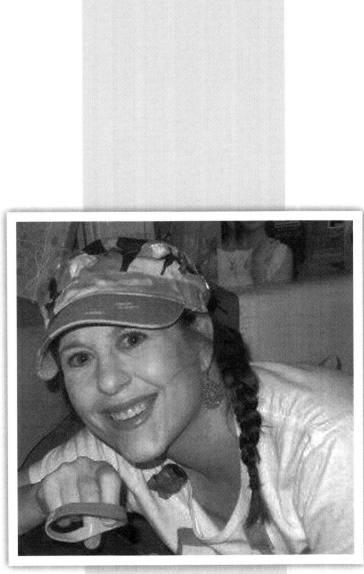

Amy Byer Shainman

BRCA1 Previvor, 43
Florida USA

My BRCA Story

2010 was a very difficult year for my family and me. However, from my experience I learned great lessons of self-worth, beauty, and empowerment. I am greater than the sum of my parts.

Like a tinted moisturizer with SPF, I am luminous, authentic, joyful, and now better protected. Like a soothing eye cream, the crow's feet around my eyes have been diminished knowing that I have drastically reduced my risk for any future "wrinkles" in my life. I have become a more solid foundation for my family, while discovering a newfound purpose to help others.

I am what is called a previvor - someone who has never had cancer but has an extraordinarily high risk for getting it. I inherited the BRCA1 gene mutation #5385 (aka #5382) from my Dad. It's one of the three founder mutations associated with people of Ashkenazi Jewish descent. I had up to an 87% chance of getting breast cancer in my lifetime and up to a 50% risk of getting ovarian cancer in my lifetime (compared to the 10% and 4% respectively of the normal population). I chose to be fierce and strong. I chose to be fearless and to conquer. I made the decision to be here for my husband, my kids, and most importantly myself. I let go of my dream of having more children and instead took on the side effects of menopause. I said good riddance to my ticking time bomb breast tissue and welcomed my new breasts with implants and minimal scars. I became my own advocate and ultimately a pioneer in my family.

The family tree on my father's side looks like a road map for hereditary female cancers. My grandmother Lillian died in 1934 at age 33 from breast cancer and what I believe was most likely ovarian cancer as well. Her mother died of breast cancer, plus several of my father's female first cousins had breast cancer. However, we only really looked at our family tree when my sister Jan got diagnosed and treated for both ovarian cancer and uterine cancer (two separate primary cancers) in the fall of 2008. It was then we learned that she carried the BRCA1 #5385 genetic mutation. We had heard of BRCA testing but simply weren't aware of what testing actually meant. We didn't realize that there had been two identified gene mutations - BRCA1 and BRCA2. Plus, we didn't know that there were many different specific mutation numbers within the BRCA1 and BRCA2 mutations.

We had no idea that if you were of Ashkenazi Jewish descent, that alone raises an eyebrow for concern. One out of every 40 Jewish people carries a mutation in the BRCA1 or BRCA2 gene. We had no knowledge that the different mutation numbers meant different things in terms of cancer risk. In addition, we learned that a BRCA gene mutation can be passed onto you from either your mother OR your father and that you have a 50% percent chance of inheriting it from that carrier. More than that, a BRCA gene mutation in a woman has also very different and significantly higher risks associated with it than if a man carries a BRCA gene mutation.

At the same time my sister was undergoing chemotherapy for ovarian cancer, my dear friend Kristin was battling triple negative breast cancer from her own BRCA1 (not Ashkenazi Jewish) Icelandic mutation. Two BRCA cancer battles were happening right in front of me altering my perspective on everything. I credit both Jan and Kristin with saving my life. Being BRCA positive put me at great risk for getting cancer, plus I had extremely dense breast tissue, which is known to "hide" cancer (it's difficult to detect breast cancers through regular mammogram screening if you have dense breasts).

For me, I saw only two choices in front of me - do nothing or do something. I could sit around with my high-risk percentages and dense breasts and wait to see if I would get a hereditary female cancer or I could have prophylactic surgeries and virtually cure myself before any issue of cancer would arise. I watched what my sister Jan and my friend Kristin were going through and I thought to myself, "Yes, I have inherited this very dangerous genetic mutation but I have been given the gift of having options to drastically reduce my cancer risk. Knowing that I can actually do something to prevent what they are going through and even avoid death - I can't just sit on this knowledge and do nothing."

The prophylactic surgeries reduced my risk for breast cancer from about 87% to about 3% and have made it so I will never get or die from ovarian cancer, although I do still carry a small risk (about 1%) for peritoneal cancer (lining of the abdomen). My view is that I simply removed the parts of me that were causing more harm than good. This philosophy was easy for me to take on since I had already been through a major surgery in 1998 to remove a benign brain tumor (acoustic neuroma), which consequently left me completely deaf in my right ear.

I am invigorated with passion and purpose. I feel a deep responsibility to share what I have learned about hereditary breast and ovarian cancer and BRCA gene mutations; compelled to pay it forward by sharing my BRCA story and spreading risk awareness to women, just like the information was given to me. I have found that a lot of women have heard of BRCA but really don't know exactly what testing positive for a gene mutation means. My decision to have preventative surgeries is what was right for me; however, it may not be right for everyone. Other options for breast cancer risk reduction include taking Tamoxifen and/or enhanced surveillance/screenings. However, there are currently no accurate ovarian cancer surveillance/screening methods. I hope that all women realize that knowing their family medical history and learning how they can stay healthy is really the most loving thing they can do for themselves and their loved ones.

How did I find out all of this information about BRCA? Most of what I have come to know about my BRCA1 genetic mutation was provided by FORCE (Facing Our Risk of Cancer Empowered) www.facingourrisk.org What is FORCE? FORCE is a nonprofit organization for women whose family history or genetic status puts them at high risk of getting ovarian and/or breast cancer, and for members of families in which risk is present. The mission of FORCE is to improve the lives of these individuals and families. I am currently the Palm Beach County, Florida outreach coordinator for FORCE. Outreach groups provide support, resources, and education. It was the June 2010 FORCE conference that provided my sister and me with invaluable information that helped us make important life-saving decisions. If there is a history of breast and/or ovarian cancer in your family, you owe it to yourself to go see a certified genetic counselor. Unlike your OB/GYN or primary care physician, a genetic counselor is trained to assess your background, deem if genetic testing is advisable for you, and then administer the test. A genetic counselor knows how to interpret the test results--which is hugely important since you will be making health decisions based on those test results. Plus, if no genetic mutation is found with testing, a genetic counselor will still be able to correctly counsel you as to what your lifetime screening and /or monitoring should be. You may still be at higher risk than the average population.

If you don't know your family medical history, start asking about it now. Knowledge is definitely power. Listen to your inner voice; if you suspect that your genes may be putting you at risk for cancer, contact a genetic counselor instead of analyzing it yourself. A genetic counselor is the best first step for someone to take because they will know how to counsel you on what to do.

My friend Kristin Hoke succumbed to her disease in June of 2010 at age 42. My husband Jon and I share our story at www.jupiterbreastcare.com in support of The Kristin Hoke Breast Health Center and because the knowledge about hereditary cancer can simply save lives.

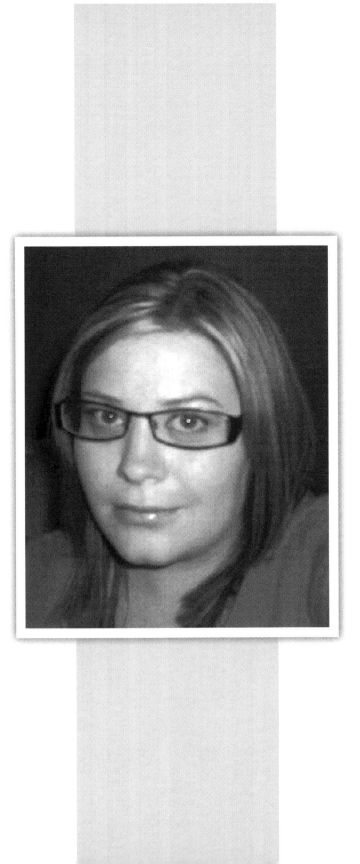

Krystal Mikita

BRCA1 Previvor, 28
Winnipeg, Manitoba CANADA

The Road Less Traveled

I can't pinpoint exactly when my journey began. I do know my story closely intertwines with my mom's.

1998 was going to be a great year. I was starting my last year of middle school and I couldn't be more thrilled. I was looking forward to finishing up and moving on to high school where I vowed to reinvent myself. About week or so into the school year I was told that my mom had been diagnosed with Stage IV ovarian cancer. I really didn't know what to think because the only thing I had heard about cancer up to that point was that people died from it. Panic and fear set in pretty quickly and I made regular visits to the guidance counselor's office. Having come from a pretty dysfunctional family my mom was the one who held us together. She was the glue of the family.

When I look back on the time my mom was sick the four years blur together for me. She spent most of that time in the hospital. Emotionally I was a mess. I was trying to deal with becoming a teenager and also watching my usual energetic mom go through so much pain. She went through surgery and chemotherapy. When her treatment wasn't working she was sent to Grand Forks, ND from our hometown in Winnipeg, Manitoba, Canada for radiation treatment. The waitlist for radiation in Winnipeg was so long and her doctors knew she didn't have that kind of time.

I tried to do normal things like have a part-time job, go to school and spend time with friends but it was a lot to handle. I suppose I was trying to maintain some normalcy because I had become the girl who had a sick mom. My peers were not very nice to me.

In the last year of my mom's life she was moved to palliative care at the hospital where she had once worked. I spent a lot of quality time with my mom that last year and learned a lot about her. We had so much fun that year. I would spend the night in her room with her and paint her nails and watch girly movies and talk until we both fell asleep. She celebrated her 39th birthday in the hospital. She had her makeup done and we had a little party for her with family and friends from church.

Shortly after her birthday she started hallucinating and was not herself. Her doctor said it was because the cancer had spread to her brain. She had told me so many times since she got sick that the only thing that kept her fighting was my brother and I. But the cancer had taken over and she couldn't fight anymore. She soon slipped into coma. We would sit with her and talk to her and deep down I knew she could hear us even when the doctors said they weren't sure she could. On June 14th we had been visiting with her and something came over me where I really felt the need to be alone with her. I asked my family to leave the room so I could have some time with her. I sat at her bedside holding her hand. I remember she always had the nicest, softest hands. I told her how strong she was and how much

I loved her. I told her that she could let go and didn't have to fight anymore. We would be okay. For the first time in a week or so she opened her eyes just slightly and said I love you too and closed them again.

June 15th my brother and I woke up in the morning to the phone ringing. It was my grandmother calling to wake us up for school. She had said my Dad went to the hospital in the middle of the night. I later found out the doctors called to inform him my mom was having very hard time breathing. I really didn't want to go to school that day but I did. Just before lunchtime I got called to the office. The principal told me that my youth leaders from church would be coming to pick me up to take me to the hospital and to wait at the front of the school. I don't think I was waiting long but it felt like an eternity until my friends arrived. Not too long after I arrived at the hospital my mom took her last breath.

I was a total mess for several years after my mom passed away. I rebelled and did things I never thought I would do. I didn't want to deal with the emotions and everything surrounding my mom's death. My family had fallen apart at the seams. I didn't begin to deal with her death until I got into a relationship with someone I felt I could trust completely. I finally let my guard down.

Shortly after that relationship ended at the age of 24 I tested positive for the BRCA1 gene mutation. At the time I had no idea what BRCA was or how the mutation could affect my life. I always had the thought of when I am diagnosed with cancer not if because I knew that there was a strong family history of it on my mom's side of the family. When I received a call out of nowhere from a genetic counselor who explained that my mom had asked her to locate my brother and me so that we could be tested I almost felt relieved.

When I met with her she told me about FORCE. I decided to test that day. I then went home and read through the message boards and other information on FORCE. I think learning as much as I could about the gene became an obsession. In 2009 I decided with the help of a counselor through the breast health center that I would have a prophylactic bilateral mastectomy with DIEP reconstruction. I saw a few different breast surgeons before I found the right fit for me and had chosen my plastic surgeon after researching about 10 or so.

While waiting for my surgery date I was constantly trying to process what was about to happen. I never doubted my decision to have surgery. But there were a lot of emotions that surfaced while preparing myself mentally for the surgery. I had lot of anger. Not anger towards a person but anger towards cancer and all it had done to my life. I saw the counselor at the breast health center frequently and we worked through all of my emotions. I began to detach myself from my breasts, which were one of the few parts of my body that I was actually comfortable with. I didn't have a large support system at the time. There were some people that were very supportive of why I was having surgery and some that thought it was a pretty drastic decision to remove my healthy breasts and go through all that recovery and future surgery.

I had surgery in June of that year and it was very sentimental to me that I was having surgery in the same month that my mom passed. I decided that I did not want anyone to come to the hospital with me. I felt like I needed to conquer this on my own. As I walked into the hospital there was that brief moment of fear where something told me to run out of the hospital. I am so glad I didn't give into that fear. I had some complications with an abscess that needed to be drained and some of the stitches not taking. The complications seem minor though in comparison to the high risk that I had.

In 2010 I was due to have revision surgery and nipple reconstruction. However I became pregnant and postponed it. Shortly after my son's first birthday I underwent revisions and nipple reconstruction. It's been about five and a half months since that surgery and I am slowly healing. It is much harder to recover when you are running after an active toddler all of the time. I have been having some issues with the nerves on my sides since revision surgery. My plastic surgeon says it is because the nerves are trying to regenerate themselves and suffering from fibromyalgia it makes the pain worse. But I am pushing through because if my mom could fight as hard as she did through all she went through I can fight through this to prevent having to fight through that.

My plan for the near future is to continue having CA-125 tests as a type of surveillance and staying on top of what is going on in my body. I know that there is no real screening for ovarian cancer. That is why my mom wasn't diagnosed until it was too late. There are so many other things that have the same symptoms that we pass them off as something else.

I plan on having an oophorectomy in my early thirties once I know for sure that I am done having children. In the past year or so I have been blessed to get to know some amazing people through the Pink Moon. We are all one big family and I am grateful for all the love and support. It is nice knowing there are people that can relate to the things that I am going through.

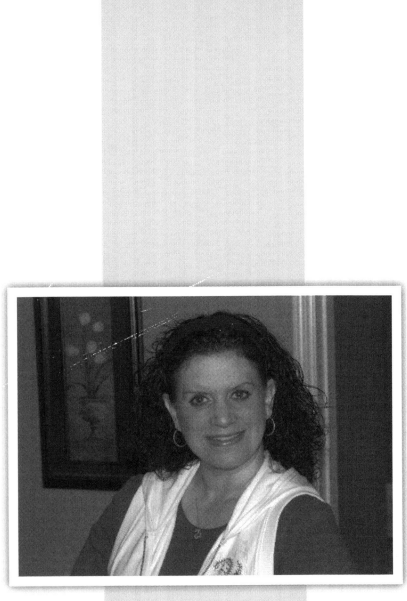

Lisa Ward

BRCA1 Previvor, 43
USA

The Gift of Love ~ My Previvor Story

My story begins with my mom who passed away from ovarian cancer in January 2008. Thankfully she had the BRCA test that would save my life. She tested positive for the BRCA1 gene.

My older sister and I decided to get tested. She went first and her result came back negative for the genetic mutation. Her result left me scared. I knew I had a 50/50 chance that I could be a carrier. As I waited for my result to come back I had a feeling it would be positive for the gene. After all my mom, aunt, grandmother and grandfather all died from cancer. All of them were on my mother's side of the family. The odds didn't look good for me. What were the chances that my sister and I would both be negative?

In March 2008 my husband and I traveled to Decatur, Alabama so I could be tested for the genetic mutation. We discussed my options and talked about the choices I would make if my results came back positive for the gene. We began planning the necessary steps we were leaning towards. Weeks later the crushing news arrived. My test results came back as I had anticipated. I was positive for the BRCA1 gene mutation. In the weeks before both my husband and I prepared for the worst and prayed for the best. We both agreed that I would move forward with preemptive surgeries. My husband said he wanted to keep me around for the rest of our lives.

My preemptive choices had been decided. I was scheduled to have a bilateral mastectomy with reconstruction and a total hysterectomy with a bilateral oophorectomy. This meant that I would be removing my breasts, uterus and ovaries. We scheduled to have my hysterectomy and oophorectomy done first. My doctors chose to do a vaginal hysterectomy and a laparoscopic oophorectomy. There was quite a bit of pain and discomfort involved in my healing, but overall it went very well. My family was there to help me whenever I needed them for anything. I was truly blessed to have them there for me every day of my recovery process.

A few months later I scheduled my bilateral mastectomy and the beginning stages of the reconstruction surgeries. Overall the surgery went well. My surgeon had my breast tissue sent off to be tested. The pathology report came back that I had cysts that were forming. Thankfully, none of them were cancerous. "THANK the LORD!!" We felt so blessed that we were able to catch this early. I felt as if I had been given a second chance at life. I had been given a gift from my mom. If my mom had not tested for the BRCA gene, I most likely would have been the next member in the family fighting for my life. My mom was my guardian angel. Had it not been for BRCA test I could have been fighting breast cancer right now. But instead, I am able to share my story of hope.

During the reconstruction portion of my mastectomy, my plastic surgeon placed expanders in my breast cavities. Over the next few months my husband and I made several trips to the surgeon's office to have my expanders filled with saline. I remember that after each fill I felt like I had an elephant sitting on my chest. I don't recall the number of visits it took for me to get my full expansion, but I do remember it being uncomfortable. Thankfully the discomfort only lasted a few days.

In February 2009 I was scheduled to have my expanders removed, in exchange for implants. My husband referred to them as bionic boobs!! I am so thankful that I have a husband that attended every doctor's appointment with me and stood beside me and supported me every step of my BRCA journey. It was not easy, but he never skipped a beat. I am filled with much love and gratitude.

In the coming years when my daughter and son are of age they too will be tested for the BRCA1 gene. My husband and I are praying they will not have to face this unfortunate fate. Thankfully for my husband and I my journey was short. If my beautiful guardian angel had not gotten tested, I am certain we would have been on a much longer journey, one that would have made me wonder if I would make it to the end.

I thank the Lord so much for allowing me the gift to be cancer free at this time and hopefully for the remainder of my life!

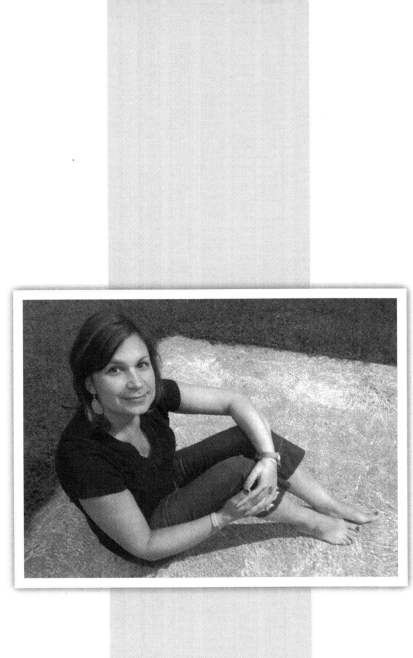

Nina Z.W.

BRCA1 Previvor
Pennsylvania USA

No Regrets

I am 41 years old. I live in West Chester, PA about 40 minutes outside of Philadelphia. I have a terrific husband, Brian. We have been married for 14 years. I have two great boys that are 10 and 8. I have been fortunate to be a stay-at-home mom. Prior to kids, I worked full time as a social worker. I hope to return to my professional career soon.

I am the youngest of six children including three sisters and two brothers. My siblings and I are first generation American born. My parents were born in the Ukraine immigrating to the United States in 1950. They divorced after 17 years of marriage when I was in elementary school. I don't ever remember them being happy.

When I was about nine my mother was diagnosed with breast cancer. She was 43. It was the 1980s. She had a radical mastectomy on the one breast. No chemo, no radiation. Seven years later she experienced stomach pains and went to see her gynecologist. Next thing I remember she was having surgery. I was 16 and had no idea what was going on. Being the baby, I was always protected by my siblings.

I distinctly remember sitting in the waiting room with my sister during her surgery. The doctors came out to talk to us in less than an hour. I said to my oldest sister, "It's not good." The doctor said, "We opened her up and had to close her up. She is full of cancer." Next was chemo. We took turns taking mom to chemo. To be honest, I hated it. She would vomit on the way home. The doctors gave her less than a year to live. She had Stage IV ovarian cancer. She lived for three years. My dear mother passed away on November 26, 1990. She held on for Thanksgiving that year. She passed a few days after. I was 19 years old and a sophomore in college. Ironically, my father died seven years and seven days later on December 3, 1997. This was four months before my wedding. It was sudden. My brother found him dead on the floor. He had a heart attack. At 27, I felt like an orphan. No mother or father to share my wedding day. Instead we displayed white roses in memory of them.

I have always worried about cancer. I would talk to my gynecologist about it. We started mammograms at 30. She also told me about BRCA testing about 10 years ago. She gave me the card to the hospital genetics counselor. I tucked it in my purse. I tucked it in the back of my head. Way back in my head. I then had my first son at 30. My OB/GYN mentioned it again at my follow up appointment. Again, notated. Then two and half years later, I had my other son. She mentions it then. I have two young boys. The last thing I am thinking about is cancer. I am on top of the world. I am in "mommy mode".

In 2009 my husband and I were discussing vasectomy or tubal ligation. Part of me just wanted my ovaries out. I knew that was what killed my mother. My husband worked with a man whose wife was a geneticist at Jefferson University Hospital. He brought home a pamphlet. There were six questions. It said if you answer yes to any of these questions, please contact our department. I answered yes to four of them. Wow! Then I mentioned to my son's pediatrician about my mother. He said, "You know there is a genetic link to breast and ovarian cancer. They do tests for that. DO IT FOR YOUR BOYS." Wow!

And then out of nowhere my oldest sister had emergency surgery to remove her ovaries. They thought she had ovarian cancer. We were all worried sick. They tested her for BRCA. She was negative. Her doctor still urged us all to get BRCA testing due to our family history. I was finally ready to test myself. On May 18, 2009 I found out I was BRCA1 positive. After the one hour counseling session, I really did not know the weight of it all. In the meantime my other two sisters were tested and they were negative.

I went home and researched the Internet and read and read. I went to my first FORCE meeting in June 2009. I felt like I had been hit by a truck. The Show and Tell just hit me like a ton of bricks. It was a lot of information to process. These are life-changing decisions. In January 6, 2010, I had a total hysterectomy and oophorectomy.

In the midst of it all a dear friend was diagnosed with breast cancer. I found out she was tested and had BRCA2. She did chemo, radiation, and had a mastectomy and oophorectomy. She was cancer free. Then in June 2011, she was having pain in her hip. She had a scan. She had liver, bone, and lung cancer.

Prior to this, I was diagnosed with another health condition. I left the BRCA world for a bit. Just trying to get out of pain, and get "healthy". My friend was doing great. Her tumors were shrinking. Then in December 2011 things took a turn for the worse. Her tumors were growing fast. My dear sweet friend passed away on January 28, 2012 on my oldest son's birthday.

This threw me into a tailspin. I jumped back into the BRCA world. Soon after I read the book <u>Beyond the Pink Moon</u> thanks to Nicki Boscia Durlester. What a fantastic book! I started the process of meeting with surgeons. Asking lots of questions.

Every year my MRI was in March. I worked myself up with worry starting in February. I had an MRI on March 26, 2012. All was clear. I had my DIEP flap surgery on May 11. I really envy the women that know right off the bat that this is what they need to do. I DID NOT WANT to do this.

I did it and I have had complications. I still have more surgery ahead. No regrets. I had to do this for my family and me. I want to live a long and healthy life.

I love all the support and positive thoughts and information shared on Beyond the Pink Moon. The Pink Moon Lovelies are all AMAZING. I can never thank them enough for all of their love and support.

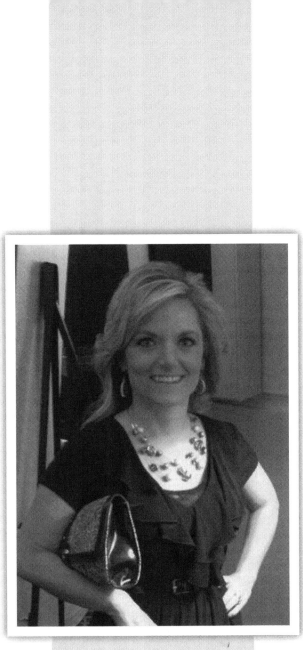

Ezzell

BRCA2 (5270del TG) Previvor, 39
St. Joseph, Missouri USA

My Endurance Creates Beauty

I had always heard of others talk about cancer, but I really never knew it to be so evil until my dad was diagnosed with lung cancer at 56. A few years before, his doctors tested him for elevated prostate levels. His levels were extremely high, but biopsies always came back negative for cancer. Now, looking back, we know his lung cancer started in his prostate. He had many rounds of chemo and radiation. Finally, the doctors gave us the bad news that there was nothing else they could do and the cancer was spreading. They gave him two months. I remember them saying "two months" and I just felt like time was physically slipping away. I went into a crying panic as I didn't know or even imagine how life would continue without this man, let alone my mother living without him. You see my dad was the rock, the breadwinner, our strength, and he was the tough guy that nothing could take him down. He was a little guy, but known to be a mighty one. A Vietnam veteran and a college football player. I never thought anything could beat my dad. Dad was tough, but to see him become weak, fragile, little, confused and in so much pain that we couldn't even move him into his bed was very traumatizing to me. Within nine months of diagnosis we lost him. I was there with my mother and brother when he took his last breath. All of us sleeping together on the floor, holding each other.

Six months later, my uncle, (my dad's brother) was diagnosed with stomach cancer. We now know it was probably pancreatic cancer and he passed within weeks. His daughter a few years later at age 35 was diagnosed with breast cancer and she was tested for the BRCA gene. She tested positive and had a double mastectomy with treatment. She is my only female cousin, so we had no idea about breast or ovarian cancer and this was a shock to us as cancer had only reared its ugly head years before with my dad. How could this be? Well, looking back, we believe my grandmother, my dad's mom, had ovarian cancer. She was trying to lose weight and could not lose her "belly". She was having other symptoms such as a full bladder, back pain and no energy. One day she went to bed and passed away. My grandfather never had an autopsy, so we don't know if she truly had ovarian cancer, but we are almost positive she did.

After my cousin tested positive, she informed me about our family history, her cancer, her result and what that meant for myself, my brother, our cousins, my aunt and uncles. I finally had the BRCA test a year after my cousin's diagnosis and her positive results. I remember thinking okay our dads had cancer and she had breast cancer, but really I don't think this will effect me. Honestly, I believed I would test negative, so much so, I forgot about my test results. I received a call one day when I was home from work and I was alone. I will never forget her saying I was BRCA2+ 5370delTG, deleterious mutation. I kept it together and grabbed a pen and paper while she was giving me statistics and information. I needed all the information I could get. I hung up the phone and just melted. Not just for me, but for my amazing children and hubby. Could my future really be wrapped in cancer? Could I leave them early and God forbid could they have the mutation too? I remember calling my mother and telling her my results. There was silence on her end of the phone and I knew she was crying. All she knew about cancer was what we experienced with Dad. I reassured her that so much could be done now and I was blessed to know I am positive, that I will take care of this for my family and myself. She did not need to worry about losing me!!

I chose to have a total hysterectomy a few months later as I knew ovarian cancer is difficult to detect and survival rates are worse than breast cancer. I was also having some issues that my grandmother had, such as bloating, back pain, and no energy. Come to find out I had a benign tumor the size of a four month pregnancy, so I am so thankful I elected to have this surgery right away. Also, I never really thought my breasts were that great, but I really didn't know how attached I was to them until after my positive results. So, I put off any idea of a mastectomy. I chose the surveillance route and some clinic trials (needle aspirations). After my last needle aspiration, I was informed my cells were rapidly changing and were atypical. I had enough of surveillance and wondering if this was it. I once heard someone explain the choice to have a PBM in this way, "If you knew a plane you were about to board had an 87% chance of crashing, would you board even if they found you soon after the crash and your survival rate would be good?" Wow, never thought of it that way.

I researched the best surgeons and started to prepare for my PBM. I remember being really strong. I get that my from dad too. However, when I felt like I couldn't handle all the emotions I was feeling leading up to surgery I would take a shower and just bawl. No one saw and no one heard me. During this time I was grieving my breasts, the loss of my womanhood, and the femininity power I would lose. One night I just couldn't hold it in anymore. I got up, went into the living room and let it all out. My hubby came in, held me and let me cry as long as I wanted. After that I was ready to go!!!

I had a nipple sparing prophylactic bilateral mastectomy with expanders on May 30, 2012. I am in the expansion process and ready to be a part of the all done club!!

I'm going to leave you with a couple of quotes I often read that have encouraged me:

The most beautiful people are those who have known defeat, known suffering, known struggle, known loss, and have found their way out of the depths. These persons have an appreciation, sensitivity, and an understanding of life that fills them with compassion, gentleness, and a deep loving concern. Beautiful people do not just happen.

Elisabeth Kübler-Ross

It is not a question of God allowing or not allowing things to happen. It is part of living. Some things we do to ourselves, other things we do to each other. Our Father knows about every bird which falls to the ground, but He does not always prevent it from falling. What are we to learn from this? That our response to what happens is more important than what happens. Here is a mystery: one man's experience drives him to curse God, while another man's identical experience drives Him to bless God. Your response to what happens is more important than what happens.

Chip Brogden

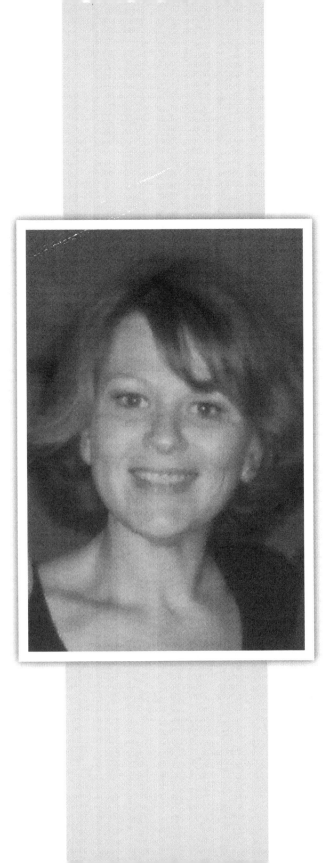

Jennifer Benedict Beaty

BRCA2 Previvor, 40
Indianapolis USA

My Story

After my grandma's ovarian cancer diagnosis, my mom, Rainy Droke, whose story is also in this book, was told about the BRCA gene. She was tested and found to be BRCA2 positive. I also tested, as did my two aunts and one cousin. All were found to be positive except one aunt.

On October 25, 2011, I had a complete hysterectomy and prophylactic bilateral mastectomy. It was a no brainer for me, as I had been with my mom when she made those same decisions and had her surgeries. I knew I would do the same, eventually.

My aunt passed away in July 2011 of lung cancer after beating breast cancer almost 10 years prior. We were told it was environmental and not hereditary, (yeah, right). My grandma died on December 16, 2011.

I wish that someone had talked with our family about this sooner! I have two daughters and am so thankful that I had this information and was able to be proactive with my health. I am also grateful that my daughters will have this information, as they get older.

I had my final surgery for nipple reconstruction and minor revisions on April 27, 2012. I am here hoping to share my story with others who know what being BRCA positive means and to help anyone with questions, if I can.

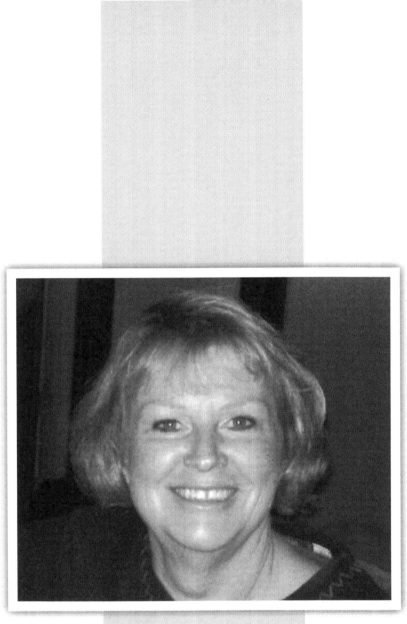

Rainy Benedict

BRCA2 Previvor, 58
Beech Groove, Indiana USA

My Life With BRCA

I am a previvor. I was with my sister ten years ago when she was told she had breast cancer. My first question to the doctor was, "Is it a genetic thing?' He kind of laughed and said it was not genetic. He blamed it on the fact that she smoked. I believed him! Wrong thing to do.

My sister went through hell with all of the treatments. She did not have reconstruction because at the time they never told her that insurance would help with the cost. I feel some doctors don't tell the whole story to patients. I'm so grateful that my doctor told me what she would do if it were she or someone in her family.

At the time my daughter, Jennifer Benedict Beaty, whose story is also in this book, was against me having anything done. I guess the old adage if it ain't broken don't fix it applies. After meeting with my doctor my daughter and I walked out knowing I had to have the prophylactic surgery.

I lost my sister in July 2011 to lung cancer after beating breast cancer ten years before. I also lost my mother in December 2011 to ovarian cancer. People need to understand this is not a wait and see game.

Let's get this message out!

C. Renée Savoie

BRCA1 Previvor, 39
Mays Landing, New Jersey USA

The Keaton Curse

"You'll be fine!" The words I hear coming from my two cousins and my sister as we just gathered for a celebration of life for my Aunt Pat. For 24 hours those words were comforting because the three of them were BRCA1 negative. We were advised by Aunt Pat to get tested because she tested positive for BRCA1 after the devastating news of Stage III ovarian cancer in 2003. It was a long battle she thought she had won, but the cancer invaded her liver and killed her at the young age of 62. I was the last of the four grandchildren to get tested.

My sister and I heard of cancer on my dad's side of the family. In 1922 my great grandmother died at the age of 41, a few days after giving birth to her 10th child who was stillborn. In our family bible it was noted that my grandmother had a "female cancer." The baby was buried with her in her loving arms. Out of 10 children, only four survived to old age. All the rest died at birth or from childhood illnesses. My grandmother was only three years old when her mother died, never really knowing her, except that cancer took her young soul at an early age.

At the age of 40, my grandmother had a partial hysterectomy. Dad and Aunt Pat were told this was customary during those days. I can't help but cry. If only my grandmother's doctors had taken her ovaries out, her suffering and death may have been avoided. In 1972 my grandmother was diagnosed with breast cancer. She was 53 it was found in her left breast. She went to the family doctor who knew very little about cancer. In the 1970s there weren't breast specialists or surgeons like we have today. She had a total mastectomy of the left breast, chemo and radiation. It was a botched operation requiring further surgery so she could have better use of her arm. She bad burns from the radiation and damage was done to the lymph nodes and muscle. Nana wore a pressure sleeve and her arm was forever painful from the fluid buildup. She was never offered reconstruction and lived her life with a sock stuffed in her bra for a makeshift breast. In 1986 my grandmother's brother died of stomach cancer and this is when the family started calling cancer, THE KEATON CURSE! Keaton was my grandmother's maiden name.

I remember sitting at the table as my grandfather would sternly but lovingly say to my grandmother, "Eat!" This went on for a year before he finally took her to the doctor. The doctor prescribed medicine for stomach issues, but it didn't work. Pop took Nana to the University of Pennsylvania in Philadelphia where they operated on her. The surgeon discovered she had ovarian cancer so bad it was flaking off and eating through her stomach wall. They closed her back up and sent her home to die. I never got to say goodbye to Nana. She didn't want us to have our last memories of her being so sick. I was 19 years old when I had to deal with death. I was so angry about

THE KEATON CURSE! In 1992 sadly Nana died of ovarian cancer at 73.

In 2001 THE KEATON CURSE struck again during my dad's routine colonoscopy. His doctor discovered rectal/colon cancer. He was 56 years old. Once again our family was back at the University of Pennsylvania hospital dealing with cancer. My dad survived. With courage and strength he gracefully beat rectal/colon cancer. I admire him greatly for that.

My dad's sister, my Aunt Pat, found out she had Stage III ovarian cancer just three years later. Her team of doctors asked her about our family history. She told them about THE KEATON CURSE. They advised her to take the "new genetic test" that was out call BRCA. Shortly after Aunt Pat was notified that she was indeed BRCA1 positive. The Keaton curse has an official medical name! Aunt Pat advised her two daughters, my sister and me to get BRCA tested. One by one Aunt Pat's two daughters and my sister tested negative.

"You'll be fine!" I hear in my head from my cousins and my sister, as I waited for my results. The day after Aunt Pat's funeral I received the call from my OB/GYN. He gave me the devastating news … I was BRCA1 positive! In that moment I felt as if I already had cancer. It didn't matter what kind. I knew the "Keaton Curse" lived within my dad and me. Those words, you'll be fine, are meaningless to someone like me, someone who feels like a ticking cancer time bomb. Walking around looking cheerful and upbeat, but inside consumed every minute with this dark cloud raining anxiety, distress and sadness.

Why me? April 2009 I found out I was BRCA1 positive. May 2009 I found myself in front of a genetic counselor at Fox Chase Cancer Center in Philadelphia trying to understand and wrap my head around what all this genetic makeup means now. I also met with a doctor who studies BRCA. The more I understood and the more I researched and lived BRCA, the more the fear turned to power within me. I have spent the last three years at Fox Chase Cancer Center every three to six months under close surveillance.

Meanwhile I got fit. I lost 85 pounds, began eating organic foods and saw a wellness doctor to keep my body alkaline to try and prevent cancer from growing. With all the research and getting healthy, nothing would take away the anxiety. It was so draining mentally and physically.

August 15, 2012, I decided to have a bilateral mastectomy with DIEP reconstruction. It took me a year of research and mental preparedness to endure this tough surgery. I could have never done it without the support of my husband, family and friends. A good support circle is a must! After six days in the hospital my husband and I left the parking garage at Fox Chase Cancer Center (FCCC). At that moment I got a rush of overwhelming emotions that are hard to describe. I cried for joy and happiness. The anxiety of getting breast cancer was completely gone! The physical pain from my surgery was nothing compared to the mental anguish I walked around with for the last three years. The dark cloud was gone and I finally felt a sense of peace within my soul that only a BRCA sister would know.

There are so many people to thank who supported me along my journey beginning with my Aunt Pat who researched our family tree and medical history. A gift she left before she died. She also advised us to get tested for BRCA, which I believe saved my life and a lot of heartache. Thank you to my team of doctors at FCCC who were great every step of the way. Thank you to my loving husband who has supported my decisions and gave me unconditional love. I deeply appreciate my family and friends who were there when I needed them most. Although my journey won't be over until I have a total hysterectomy, I feel so strong that I was able to endure all of this. I want to get the word out about BRCA to educate others on the importance of their family medical history and to be proactive with their health. Do not live in fear of cancer. Research it, educate yourselves, and know the warning signs because knowledge is power!

IN LOVING MEMORY OF:
Catherine (Weber) Keaton
06/05/1883- 05/02/1922
(female cancer)
Regina (Keaton) Wuest
01/03/1919- 10/14/1992
(breast, ovarian, stomach cancers)
Russell Keaton
01/23/1915- 11/06/1986
(stomach cancer)
Patricia (Wuest) Robinson
12/13/1946- 03/29/2009
(ovarian, liver cancer)

SURVIVOR:
Russell Wuest
(rectal/colon cancer)

PREVIVIOR:
Renée (Wuest) Savoie
(prophylactic bilateral mastectomy with DIEP reconstruction)

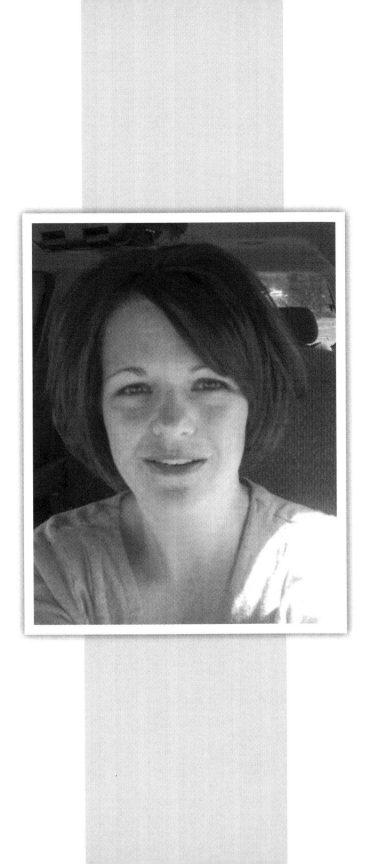

Tara Wiser Beirens

BRCA1 Previvor, 37
Pasco, Washington USA

My Journey

As long as I can remember my mom struggled. She didn't know how to be a parent. Her mother died when she was three years old and my grandpa didn't know what to do with seven young children. So he farmed them out to family or whoever would take them. I don't know much about my mom's side of the family. I met three out of her six siblings. Although my grandfather was an alcoholic, he was my savior. I loved him more than anything. My grandmother was diagnosed at the age of 36 with ovarian cancer and passed away at 38. She was too young to die. Although my mom was only three she remembered when my grandmother went into the hospital and never came out. She became pregnant with my mother.

Growing up wasn't easy for me. My mother loved us the best way she could. She buried her pain and anger in alcohol and drugs. When times were good they were great and when they were bad they were the worst. As I got older it became more difficult to be close to my mom. As an adult our relationship was extremely strained. We didn't talk for years at a time. She always expected something. I remember when she called me in 1998 to tell me my aunt was diagnosed with ovarian cancer. She was convinced it was genetic. I went to my doctor at the time and discussed the possibility that my aunt's ovarian cancer was hereditary. She didn't think it was. She believed it was due to the fact that my aunt did not take good care of herself. My aunt subsequently had chemo and was cancer free for 13 years.

On a Sunday in January in 2008 I received a call from my mom. I hated when she called me. I hated letting her in. She never did anything without it benefiting her in some way. I hadn't seen her in two years and only talked to her a handful of times. She hadn't even met my youngest daughter, Abbigal. I had enough of the ups and downs in our relationship. No matter how hard I tried I would never be good enough in her eyes. I desperately wanted a mom I could share my life with and not be judged or ridiculed for my faults. Unfortunately, I knew that would never happen. Mom said she had gone to the emergency room for a pain in her side. They did an MRI and found a large mass. She was pretty sure it was ovarian cancer. The doctors wouldn't say what it was. They referred her to an oncologist in Spokane, Washington. All she said was, "You're done having kids. You need to have everything removed now." I told her I wasn't going to do something that drastic if I didn't have to. I assured her I would see my doctors. I did this because I was convinced the cancer was caused by something more than poor lifestyle choices and bad habits. I felt it was hereditary even though years before the doctor said it wasn't.

My mom saw a specialist in Spokane who confirmed it was ovarian cancer. She suggested genetic counseling, but my mom refused. Her excuse was that her insurance would not pay for it. Looking back I think she was scared. My mother had surgery. Her final pathology showed she had Stage IV ovarian cancer. She had chemo and had allergic reactions, so her doctors tried different protocols.

In the meantime I went to my doctors to ask about my risk. They referred me to a genetic counselor who wanted my mom or my aunt to have the BRCA testing. My mom refused. She wouldn't do it even with my begging and pleading. Nor would my aunt. I couldn't understand why my mom wouldn't do it for the benefit of her children and grandchildren. She wouldn't even speak to a genetic counselor. She already believed it was genetic and felt I should have everything removed. The hardest part was telling my genetic counselor my mother said no. Although surprised, she recommended giving my mom some time hoping she might change her mind. I waited a whole year. My mom never changed her mind.

In February 2009 my genetic counselor called and said it was time for me to do something. We set up a meeting to get the testing done. I wasn't going to wait any longer for cancer to get me too. I met with her and had my blood tested for the BRCA mutation. Deep in my soul I knew I had the gene. About three weeks after I had the test I started having some cramps and could not find my IUD. My gynecologist did an ultrasound and found a seven-centimeter mass on my right ovary. It felt like the walls were caving in. I was 34 years old. This could not be happening to me. No matter how much they told me it was benign I couldn't help but worry. That was on a Wednesday. By Friday I was in surgery having the whole ovary removed. Thankfully my results were benign. No cancer. Phew! What was a relief! When I called my genetic counselor to tell her about the cyst she told me my BRCA test results were back. We set up an appointment to discuss the results. She said she was glad I did the test. Her exact words were, "We would have been screening for the wrong gene." She also told me she was shocked about the results. My heart sank. Even though deep down I knew I had the BRCA mutation, I didn't want to believe it. I was BRCA1. She thought I would be BRCA2. I remember feeling like I couldn't breathe.

My geneticist said she would contact my insurance provider to set up appointments for me to determine breast reconstruction options. We talked about what the results meant and what my risk factor was at my age. She kept repeating that nothing had to be done until I was 40 since my risk did not increase until then. She also told me not to allow anyone to bully me into doing it any sooner. I left her office in a daze. When I finally reached my husband to tell I him my results, he asked how I was doing. I was a mess. He reassured me it was all going to work out. He would love me no matter what. After speaking to him I called my mom to tell her I was positive. She told me I was wrong since we did not have breast cancer in our family. I didn't feel like arguing with her. I just restated what I was told and left it at that. I knew I wasn't going to get through to her. She was in denial. I got her address, my cousin's address and sent copies of my result to each of them. I told my brother he should get tested also. But I don't think he took me seriously. He has not been tested or talked with a doctor about it. None of my siblings have been tested to this day. It makes me sad to think they are not taking it seriously. But then again it is their choice.

So the whirlwind started when I had my first mammogram a week later. I started doing research. I think I looked at about 100 pictures of different breast surgeries. I even made my husband look. I was so worried he wouldn't find me sexy anymore, that he would never be able to touch me. He is really squeamish about that kind of stuff. We both agreed if I were to have the surgeries it would be the DIEP tram flap.

My genetic counselor talked to my insurance company and got referrals for three doctors in Seattle, Washington. She was able to set up appointments with them all on the same day. I met with a breast surgeon, an oncologist and an OB/GYN that specialized in ovarian cancer. I was pretty strong for the first two appointments. My last appointment was with the OB/GYN. I remember all went well until he got to what his recommendations were. He told me that they deduct 5 to 10 years from the age of the youngest person who died from ovarian cancer in a family. Based on my family history the doctor told me I was already at risk. I was 34 years old. How could this be happening to me? He told me that prophylactic surgery was my best option. He asked if my husband and I wanted more children knowing we had three girls and a boy. My husband and I had been talking about what we would do if I were told to have the surgery soon. He wanted to try for another boy. The OB/GYN told us we had six months to decide and to get pregnant.

My new worry was what if I don't get pregnant. What if I can't give my husband another boy? My husband assured me that it was in God's hands and if He wanted us to have another child we would get pregnant. After four months I still wasn't pregnant. I started to panic. I started to track my ovulation. I knew I didn't want to wait any longer than six months, but I also knew I would regret not having another child. Shortly after I found out I was pregnant. I don't think I could have gone through with any of the procedures if I had not gotten pregnant. My husband and I were excited but anxious to find out what we were having. Hoping for a boy, but unsure that would happen again. I also was told the pregnancy weight would help with the surgeries. I am not a very big person so any help getting fat was a plus.

During this time I hadn't spoken much to my mother. In July 2009 I received a call from my mom's boyfriend encouraging me to call her. I knew in December 2008 she was told she had liver cancer. The doctors tried radiation treatment, but her liver did not do well. They said they could not do any other treatment and she wasn't eligible for a transplant because of the ovarian cancer. When I called she told me she had a year to live. She was going to fight and win, but I knew that wasn't the case. According to her boyfriend she had a couple of months.

We went to see my mom shortly thereafter. When I told her I was pregnant she was sad but confident she would still be around for the delivery. I knew when I saw her it was only a matter of time. We talked and said we were sorry. I wish I had been a better daughter and tried harder to be closer to her. I know, however that no matter how hard I tried it would not have made a difference. It wasn't my fault we weren't close. We stayed an hour. She was tired and I knew having us there was exhausting. I called my brother and told him he needed to visit her. When he showed up the following day mom was unresponsive. He called 911 and she was rushed to the hospital. I should have just packed up right then but I didn't. My brother called an hour later and said it was time. I quickly packed some clothes and along with three of my children headed out the door. When I arrived at the hospital, everyone was there including my cousins, friends, and family. I looked at my mom lying in her bed. Her spirit was gone. She was just a shell. I am so glad I was able to talk to her before she died. After that it was a whirlwind of arrangements. Trying to find the best way to celebrate her life without upsetting anyone and making it something she would have wanted. She was cremated. We took half of my mother's ashes and poured them into the Snake River. The other half was placed in a plot so we could go and visit her. When I visit her I will go to the river. That was her favorite place to be. That is where her spirit is. My mother was finally free.

Life went on. I found out I was having a baby boy. On March 6, 2010 at 2 a.m. Gabriel Henry Matthew Beirens was born. He was 6 lbs 12 oz and 21 inches long. I was only able to breastfeed Gabe for three months. I had to stop because of the approaching prophylactic bilateral mastectomy (PBM) with DIEP reconstruction I had planned for September. It was one of the hardest things I ever had to do. But, what a miracle it is to have children and we had been blessed with five.

September rolled around quickly. I had to get through all of the preoperative appointments and organize everything at home before my surgeries. On September 20th I had my PBM. A week later on September 27th I had the DIEP Tram Flap. It has been a long two years. I am almost finished with my reconstruction. There are only minor revisions to do. I recently had my nipple reconstruction and areola tattoos done. I am so lucky I only had minor complications along the way. I knew the road was going to be trying, but I wouldn't change it for the world. I will be here to watch my children graduate from homeschool, college, get married and have grandkids. Most of all I will grow old with my soulmate. I know I wouldn't be where I am today if it wasn't for his strength. Thank you, Michael.

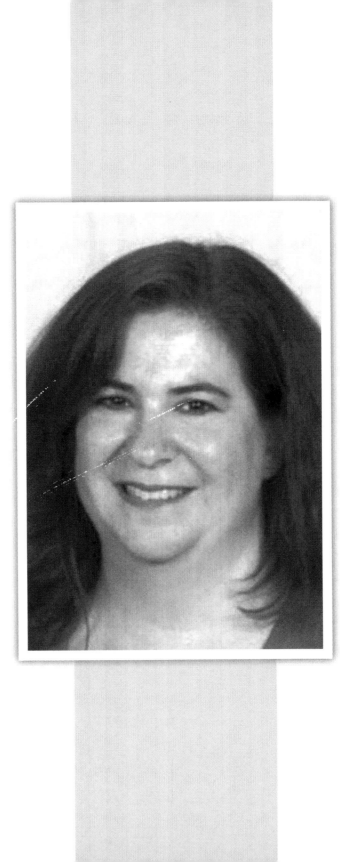

Jessica Shaw Hirshorn

BRCA2 Previvor
Scottsdale, Arizona USA

What My Father Never Knew

According to at least one research study my story starts 29 generations ago, perhaps in Spain around the time of the Spanish Inquisition with some unknown ancestor that for some unknown reason developed a mutation or spelling error on their 13 chromosome leaving out the "T." My exact mutation is 6174delT, which is considered BRCA2 and a founder mutation. If you have this mutation we have common ancestors.

My family never could spell very well, so the fact that my DNA has a spelling error in it should be of no surprise to anyone. From generation to generation this error was passed down, mothers dying at young ages for unexplained reasons. Although I don't know the history of my family going back 29 generations I do know the history going back five generations and that is the story that I would like to tell.

My great-great grandmother Judith Turkinovitch lived in the Jewish shtetl of Stolin, which is a border town not too far from Pinsk.

It is located in what today is known as Belarus, but at times was part of Russia, Poland, Ukraine and Lithuania. I imagine Stolin being something like Anatevka in Fiddler on the Roof.

I don't know exactly how old Judith was at the time of her death or what year it was, but it was sometime around the turn of the 20th century and she was in her forties. I also don't know her official cause of death, but I can surmise that it was most likely cancer related. However, I do know that she left behind a husband, Solomon and four children Jacob, Zelig, Sarah and Moishe.

Solomon came from a fairly wealthy family that was in the process of sending family members to the United States. As it was not the fashion for widowed men to live and raise children on their own it was arranged by the local yenta (matchmaker) that he would remarry to Hana Rubin who was also a widow with four children (Joseph, Rebecca, Samuel and Jack). As the story goes, Hana had the looks and Solomon had the money. Hana agreed to marry Solomon on the condition that he also send her children to live in America. So it was decided that Hana and Solomon would marry and slowly send their children to America. In 1902 stepbrother and sister Sarah and Joseph journeyed from Stolin by horse and buggy to Antwerp where they caught a boat to America.

Upon arriving in America an Aunt of Sarah's suggested that Sarah and Joseph marry each other. So in other words my great-grandparents were stepbrother and sister. Sarah and Joseph first lived in Philadelphia, PA and had four children Julia, Frances, Nathan and Vivian, but later moved to Chicago. In 1927 their son Nathan disappeared and was never heard from again. I sometimes wonder what happened to Nathan? My Grand Aunt Vivian says that her mother died of a broken heart devastated by Nathan's disappearance. Sarah's death certificate however states that at age 48 in 1928 Sarah died of breast cancer with contributory gall bladder and colon cancer.

I often think about Sarah and wonder what she must have been like. Did she look like me? Did she have my auburn hair like her daughters Frances and Vivian? I was fortunate to locate her grave that has gone forgotten and uncared for years. It is located in a section of a Chicago cemetery that is all single graves and not near any other family relatives. After giving it some thought I decided to pay for the care of her grave for at least a year. I figured that after all these years of being neglected and forgotten it was the least that I could do for my BRCA ancestor.

Two of Sarah's daughters were Frances and Vivian. Frances was my Grandmother and Vivian was my Grand Aunt, but took on the role of Grandmother after Frances died. Frances developed breast cancer in her fifties, but didn't die of it. Instead she died of a heart attack when she was in her seventies in 1975. Because I was so young when she died my memories of her are limited, but my Dad has always told me that I remind him of her. I look a lot like her and at least according to my father our personalities are similar. I sometimes wonder if along with genetic mutations, personalities can be inherited. After Frances died her sister Vivian took on the role of Grandmother. Vivian never had her own biological children; instead she adopted two children from Costa Rica. She was unable to have children because she had some type of growth on her ovaries and had to have them removed. Vivian lived a long and healthy life and died a few years ago at age 89. She was one of the most intelligent and inspiring women that I have ever met. She never had cancer and I don't know if that is because she did not have the BRCA mutation or if it was because she had her ovaries removed thus reducing her estrogen levels. I also don't know if the growth on her ovaries was cancerous or not.

I remember my father first showing me a lump that had developed on his nipple and talking about how it might be skin cancer and encouraging him go see a dermatologist. When the biopsy results first came back that he had breast cancer he was in disbelief. How can men get breast cancer, he thought to himself. He hated the color pink! He did Internet search after search on male breast cancer, all along wondering why him. Of course if he only knew what I know now. It wasn't something that he did. It wasn't his eating habits or any other environmental factors; it was because of a spelling error in his DNA that he was born with! He never knew about BRCA or what a genetic mutation was and really wasn't even aware of the history of breast cancer in his family.

He elected to have a mastectomy on his cancerous breast and had radiation. After being declared cancer free he thought that he had beat it until one day in 2006 when he again found a lump, this time under his arm. He was told that his odds of surviving were fairly good and that with chemotherapy he could live into his eighties (he was then 71), so he decided to go ahead and endure the chemo and had a port put in for the chemotherapy.

Unfortunately, later that evening he wasn't feeling very well and called me and asked me to take him to the emergency room. I have to admit that I wasn't very focused on him and was worrying instead about some trauma at work. The emergency room doctor was an idiot and was unable to figure out why he wasn't feeling well (despite the fact that we told him that my Dad had just had a port put in for chemo, his pains and his fever) and sent my Dad home without antibiotics. The next morning with a raging fever my father was rushed to the hospital. He spent the next month in the ICU with a MRSA infection that had settled in his heart ventricle. The MRSA severely weakened his heart causing him to go into congestive heart failure several times. This was very traumatic for me because I was present several times when his heart failed.

After being in the ICU and hospital for over a month his days and nights were flipped around and he grew disoriented and wanted to go home. He just wanted to go home so he demanded release from the hospital. But just because he was going home didn't mean that he was going to cease treatment and give up. We turned his living room into a hospital and each of us became nurses taking turns caring for him and giving him his meds. Unfortunately, one day my father stood up too fast and this caused him to once again go into congestive heart failure and this time there was no emergency room doctors or crash cart. My father died April 10th, 2006 of breast cancer/ MRSA and congestive heart failure. I was fortunate to be with him when he took his last gasp for air and was the last person that he saw before he died.

A few years after my father passed away a friend of mine who has a BRCA mutation told me about the genetic test and talked me into being tested. I knew that it was going to come back saying that I had the mutation, so when it did it wasn't much of a surprise. It took a few years after that for my siblings to be tested, but they both eventually were tested. My sister does not have the mutation, but my brother does.

Of course now that I knew that I had the mutation I had to decide what to do with this information. At the time I was a single mom who was caring for a terminally ill mother. I have since remarried to a wonderful man. My mother's liver disease was also genetically linked, but thankfully I did not inherit that! My life was very stressful and it seemed like every other day brought a new trauma and problem to solve. I put off addressing my BRCA diagnosis, electing instead to simply do bi-yearly screenings. This went on for four years! Yes, it took me four years to come up with a game plan. But eventually I decided to have a prophylactic bilateral mastectomy (PBM) with reconstruction and a hysterectomy. I had the PBM in December of 2011 and recently had my exchange. They had to do my PBM like a breast reduction taking away a lot of skin because I was pretty large and saggy pre-surgery. In any case, I am happy to finally have my expanders out and am hopeful that my breasts will eventually look good. Meanwhile I keep putting off having the hysterectomy because I have no real desire to be thrown into menopause within 24 hours. I really wish that there was a good way to screen for ovarian cancer so that I wouldn't have to have this surgery. However, since there is no good way to screen for ovarian cancer, I am going to have my hysterectomy this December.

I feel grateful that I have the knowledge and access to first class medical care needed to change my destiny. I have always felt that I would die at a young age. I am not sure where this feeling came from, but lately I have started to think that perhaps I am going to change my fate and break the cancer cycle. My goal is to live until my 80s having been able to watch my daughter and future grandchildren grow up. I am doing everything within my ability to achieve this goal and live a cancer free life. Hopefully sometime in the near future a vaccine or other cancer cure will be developed.

With my BRCA diagnosis and with the passing of both of my parents I have developed a strong interest in genealogy and want to trace the history of the BRCA2 6174delT mutation in my family and in general. If you have this same mutation and know your family history, please email me. I would love to be able to eventually trace it back 29 generations and learn the history of the gene!

With love and gratitude to the Pink Moon Lovelies.

Jessica Hirshorn jessicahirshorn@hotmail.com

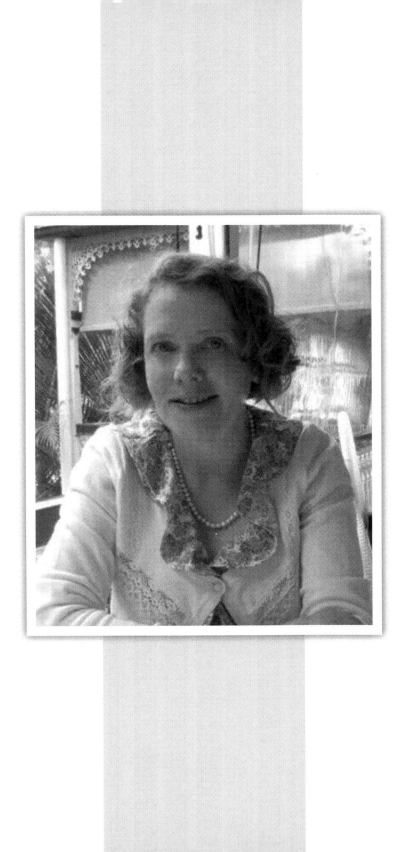

Edel Taylor

BRCA1 Previvor
Perth Western Australia, AUSTRALIA

My Story... So Far

My first memory was my 2nd birthday and being minded by my Nan and Pop as my mum was in hospital recovering from surgery for breast cancer. I clearly remember my dad bringing me my present, a shape sorter in the shape of a red British mailbox and plunking it on the floor in front of me. I was preoccupied trying to find the hole for the round shape. I had no idea that my mother was in hospital recovering from breast surgery.

I have a vague memory of visiting my mother in hospital at the time and I knew even at that age she was very sick. My mother had a radical mastectomy and removal of lymph nodes for breast cancer in the left breast. She survived but she had bad radiation burns on her skin and suffered terribly from lymphedema and cellulitis. Her left arm was permanently swollen afterwards and she always wore a compression bandage as a result.

I also recall going with mum in the pram to her follow-up radiation treatment and I remember the big machine they put her into. A young child sees their life as normal and I thought it was very normal to have a mother with a crater on her left side where her breast used to be and a swollen left arm from the lymphedema.

There was no such thing as reconstruction back then. My mother had a cloth boob that she wore and I think she suffered a huge loss in self-confidence following the surgery never wearing anything that might reveal her secret. The family history of the breast and ovarian cancer had not been pieced together and my mother assumed that her lifestyle had caused it. She straightaway gave up smoking and went on a complete lifestyle and diet change. She went on a healthy food regime, which included multitudes of vitamin pills, sea salt and kelp. You name it, we ate it or took it!! Vitamin C, cod liver oil, kelp, multivitamins, and vitamin E.

School lunches were vegemite and walnut sandwiches, which is not what the average 8-year-old loves finding in their lunchbox. We were the healthiest family in the southern hemisphere when I was growing up. This was way before any of this was fashionable.

As my mother had the radical mastectomy when I was two, she could not have anymore children and I went from being the first born to the only child until they adopted two boys, Tom and Frank two years later. My Nan and Pop and my aunt Margaret took over the care of me whilst my mother was sick and I lived with them for months when I was two. I became very close to them and Auntie Marg became like a second mother. She took me in to work with her at the hospital where she worked as a physio and I was made useful by singing to the other physios and the patients in exchange for milk coffee biscuits. Auntie Marg was always taking me to the movies and organizing special Christmas presents. One year I was presented with a magnificent dollhouse that one of her physio patients had made. It was so lovely to have this special aunt in my life.

When I was 11 Auntie Marg became ill overseas at a physio conference. The doctors in London knew her fate and told her to return to Australia as soon as possible for further treatment. Her trip was abruptly curtailed and she returned immediately to Australia. She went into hospital for surgery the day after her return home. Unfortunately they found that she had bilateral breast cancer that had spread to her liver and sadly was inoperable. I remember this time like yesterday.

She was a strong, extremely healthy looking woman and overnight she became a frail, extremely sick looking woman. She only lived two months after the diagnosis and it was a very raw time. I remember the unbearable pain she suffered and how she couldn't keep any food down. I remember my Auntie Mon (Auntie Marg's sister), a trained nurse having to care for her at home and how hard that was. I remember my mother making her fruit salad, the only thing she could eat and taking it to her every day. I remember mum getting us to make cassette tapes of us singing and playing our instruments to brighten her days and my mother couldn't bear me playing any sad music on the piano or cello at the time. I remember I was learning a funeral march by Chopin on the piano and my mother could not bear me practicing it at all. Sadly Auntie Margaret passed away two months after diagnosis at the age of 46. I was and still am devastated by this, as she was my favorite aunt.

When I was 14 my mother's sister Barbara was also diagnosed with breast cancer when her 6th child was a baby. This was particularly hard for her as Uncle Brian was a Federal Senator and was away in Canberra for the sittings of parliament quite a lot. She had breast cancer that had spread to her lungs and brain. Auntie Mon rallied to help and the rest of the family did as well as they had always been close. Auntie Barb fought this bravely but sadly she passed away a few years later, which was devastating for my cousins losing their beloved mother.

My mother survived the breast cancer well with no relapses throughout my childhood. However she became ill suddenly in 1991 at the same time I was to give birth to my daughter, Jacqui. She was in and out of hospital for tests and I had no idea what was going on as I wasn't told - she didn't want me to know and worry. However, a friend who visited me in hospital following Jacqui's birth did tell me my mother had "cancer cells" so I knew something was up. It turned out she had a second primary cancer - advanced ovarian cancer. It was called ovarian cancer but it was likely to have been primary peritoneal cancer. She was put on the drug Tamoxifen that unfortunately made her very ill. She often didn't take this drug because it made her so sick.

I had planned to go Christmas shopping with her on the December 17, 1991, but she rang me the night before to say she couldn't go, as she wasn't well enough. I thought she must be quite unwell as my mother was never too sick to go shopping. I will never forget the phone call I received from my dad the following morning to say that she had died suddenly. It was so sudden I simply didn't believe him, but unfortunately it was very true. She had suffered a pulmonary embolism, which was attributed to the drug Tamoxifen. A serious side effect of this drug is blood clots. I lost my mother suddenly one week before Christmas 1991 - the funeral being almost on Christmas Eve.

This was a devastating loss for a young mother with a seven-month-old baby. My children have grown up never knowing a grandmother on either side of the family as my husband Johnny's mother and father split up when he was three and he has never seen his mother since. She never made contact, which was sad so I have never met my mother-in-law. Despite this we have continued to forward photos of our children to her in Sydney over the years and when Johnny became very ill in early 2009, we did get a letter from her out of the blue so we know she appreciated us keeping in touch.

The genetic pattern became very clear when my first cousins developed breast cancer at a young age as well. In 1993, my 32-year-old cousin Marianne went to the doctor about a lump in her breast and was told it was a blocked duct as she was breast-feeding. She fought to get treatment for this.

She went back and forth to the doctors for months before she was even offered a scan. They said she was too young for breast cancer. Unfortunately the scans confirmed the worst. She had a very aggressive form of breast cancer, which had already spread. She had chemo and put up an enormous fight and for a time it looked like she might beat it. Unfortunately in 1998, she went downhill and died at the age of 38 leaving three young children.

Marianne's mother, Auntie Cath (my mother's sister) has since tested negative to the BRCA1 gene, which opens up a lot of questions because the gene is passed down through my mother's side. As Marianne's cancer presented in the same way as my other relatives that would have had the gene also, and she developed the cancer at 32, it would be very surprising if she didn't have the gene yet her mother tested negative to the gene test. It makes me wonder whether the gene test result was inaccurate or if we actually have more than one mutation in the family. I think the latter is very possible.

Around the same time another cousin, Gemma, the daughter of my Auntie Barb, was diagnosed with breast cancer at the age of 34. She also got the run around as well because she was so young, but she demanded scans and eventually got the surgery. Gemma has survived two lots of breast cancer and is doing really well. She is a true survivor.

In 2003, my mother's sister Mary became ill suddenly. Tests confirmed she had advanced Stage III ovarian cancer. She was a strong woman who was a trained nurse and vet who worked tirelessly with disabled children teaching them to ride horses with the Riding for the Disabled. Mary had survived a heart attack several years earlier but cancer is vicious and unfortunately Auntie Mary died in February 2004.

Around the same time as Auntie Mary's death another cousin Linda was diagnosed with breast cancer at 42 and underwent treatment. Routine tests confirmed that she had ovarian cancer so she needed a radical hysterectomy as well. Amazingly this cousin tested negative to the BRCA1 gene (the gene identified in our family) and also negative to BRCA2 gene. This is extraordinary to have two primary cancers at age 42 and to come from a BRCA family, but to test negative to the gene. No one seems to be able to explain that. Auntie Cath's (mother of Marianne who died at of cancer at 38) negative result is really odd as well. There has been a lot of interest in my family from cancer researchers due to the very unusual patterns.

Following on from this, another cousin Mary, the sister to Gemma and daughter of my Auntie Barb, developed an aggressive form of breast cancer in 2008 at 42. She underwent a bilateral mastectomy and removal of lymph nodes, which was followed by chemotherapy. Luckily this cousin, who tested positive to the BRCA1 gene, is doing really well.

I have always had very dense breasts and gynecological symptoms but they have always been benign. My first mammogram at the age of 25 noted that I had very dense breasts predisposed to breast cancer. I knew then that the cancer must be genetic even though the gene was still not known about. I was forever being called back to be rescanned and I had a particularly frightening experience in 2002 that very nearly put me off further scans for life which would have been fatal. A routine ultrasound showed that the there were significant changes in the left breast compared to the previous scan. I remember waiting forever whilst they compared the scans and decided what they would do. They sent me for a core biopsy that very afternoon. They did 16 biopsies of a particular area of the breast and I felt like I was a goner for sure given the family history! Then there was the wait for several days for the results - which seemed like an eternity. They came back benign. After this experience I should have been very vigilant, but it had the opposite effect. I was so frightened after that I was too scared to go back for scans. I fell out of the system for a couple of years and I think the next scan was in 2005, which was normal. Again I fell out of the system and wasn't scanned again until 2009.

I had a serious work accident in 2009 and I was under constant medical care and the family history came out in the open in a very big way and I was referred for gene testing and further surveillance. I fell down a flight of stairs at work with my cello landing on my left arm and the left side of my neck collecting multiple injuries including direct trauma to the left ulnar nerve resulting in paralysis in the left hand, fractured left elbow, fractured left ankle, dislocation to the left kneecap, a left shoulder injury and damage to several discs in the spinal cord as well. As a professional cellist the left hand paralysis has been absolutely devastating and life changing.

The doctors treating me for this asked me if there were any health issues in the family and I said, "Just some cancer." Apart from that I was extremely healthy. I hadn't been to the doctor in five years and my records had been archived. They wanted to know more and a massive can of worms was opened up!

The list was extensive:

- My mother had breast and ovarian cancer - two separate primaries.
- Auntie Barb (mother's sister): breast cancer
- Auntie Marg (mother's sister): bilateral breast cancer - spread to liver
- Auntie Mary (mother's sister): ovarian cancer
- Marianne (1st cousin daughter of mother's sister Cath) - breast cancer
- Linda (1st cousin - daughter of mother's brother Mick) breast and ovarian cancer - negative for BRCA1 mutation
- Gemma (1st cousin - daughter of mother's sister Barbara) - breast cancer twice, BRCA1
- Mary (1st cousin - daughter of mother's sister Barbara) - breast cancer, BRCA1
- Jessica (daughter of mother's sister Mary) - ovarian and breast cancer
- Great Aunt Barbara: breast cancer
- 2nd cousin Coraley: breast cancer

This was the tip of the iceberg, as the cancer in the extended family on my mother's side hasn't really been fully investigated yet!

My gynecologist/oncologist told me it was one of the worst family histories of breast/ovarian cancer he had ever seen.

I was referred to Genetics WA who referred me for a gene test for the BRCA1 gene mutation in March 2010, as this mutation had been identified in my family in my cousins Gemma and Mary. My result came back in May 2010. Positive for the BRCA1 gene mutation as well. The mutation was the 68_69delAG /185delAG mutation which is one of the founder mutations.

A pedigree mutant. This gene mutation must come from my mother's maternal family (Bellinger side) from the pattern of cancer in the family. My mutation has been traced back to 2000 years ago to a handful of people in Israel.

It is quite remarkable that they can trace genes back like that and even more remarkable that I have a gene that can be traced back that far. I have been fascinated by my genetic history ever since. I have had gynecological symptoms all my life starting with surgery at age 20 for an ovarian cyst. I have had lifelong problems with bleeding and in 2006 I was hospitalized as I was hemorrhaging. They thought that I must be pregnant and miscarrying. I wasn't. I had precancerous polyps instead. I underwent a hysteroscopy in September 2009 and had the precancerous polyps removed. The specialist wanted to do the full hysterectomy ASAP but it had to be postponed twice due to injuries from an accident. He thought it wouldn't matter whether I tested positive or negative. I needed the surgery all the same because with my family history testing negative meant nothing.

I underwent a total hysterectomy and removal of the ovaries in July 2010 at the recommendation of my specialist. Luckily it was keyhole surgery so I recovered quickly and I have miraculously had no side effects from the surgery. I've had no menopausal symptoms at all which is extraordinary.

I was then referred to a breast surgeon who immediately recommended a prophylactic bilateral mastectomy due to my massive family history, my BRCA1 positive status, my very dense breast and my long history of benign breast lumps. She told me I would get breast cancer in the next couple of years. My last scans from October 2011 showed further changes, which my specialist was concerned about. She said she couldn't rule out that it was malignant, but if so it would only be early breast cancer. Well that was cheery news!!

I therefore underwent the prophylactic bilateral mastectomy in November 24, 2011. We don't celebrate Thanksgiving Day in Australia but on this Thanksgiving Day I was definitely giving thanks!! The pathology was clear but my decision was definitely the right one. I had defied my destiny. I am quite elated that I had the surgery just in time and outsmarted the beast.

I took part in a world trial of air expanders and I had metal air canisters inserted into my chest, which are pumped up on a daily basis with air. The exchange to implant is faster with this new method and it is less invasive than the saline implants, as there are no injections. However, all expanders are barbaric I reckon. I called them my "bocce balls." I'm so pleased with the result though.

My plastic surgeon is an outstanding craftsman and even though I lost my nipples it actually looks like I still have them from the way he did the reconstruction. Quite amazing! I had the exchange on the March 1, 2012 and I had the nipple reconstruction September 19, 2012, which gave me some closure to the whole experience. I am now planning the tattooing. I think I had better not tell my 18-year-old son that as he said he wanted a tattoo and I told him, "Over my dead body you will!" I will look like a hypocrite.

Currently another cousin, Jessica, is battling advanced ovarian and breast cancer at the age of 44. She has a four-year-old boy and is single. She is such an amazingly strong woman. Her prognosis was poor, but she is responding remarkably well to the chemo treatment, some of the tumors have disappeared altogether, which is miraculous! I continue to hope and pray that she is spared for little Lachlan's sake.

The question still remains whether my kids Jacqui, 21 and Charlie, 18 have the gene as well. Jacqui is having the test later this year and she is quite philosophical about it all and is not daunted or worried by a positive result. She knows that she can make choices to change her destiny. Hopefully, there is a vaccination just around the corner, which would mean no preventative surgeries. That would be awesome!!

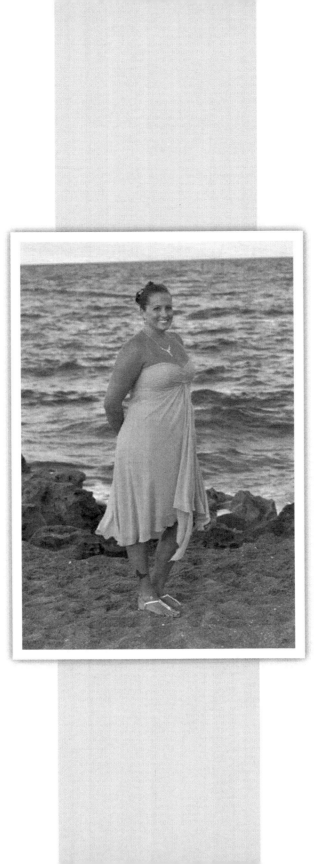

Jessica Tyson

BRCA1 Previvor, 33
Jupiter, Florida USA

Everything Happens For A Reason

My story begins when I was seven years old and lost my mother to breast cancer. I remember the last day I saw her. My dad and step mom had taken my brother, who was 12, my sister who was 16 and I to the hospital to spend time with her. Up until that day I had not been to visit her. Looking back now my dad and step mom must have known it was her last day and wanted me to see her. I don't physically remember seeing her but I do remember going to the hospital, all of us leaving her room and my mother asking my step mom to stay behind to talk to her.

On the way home from the hospital the car was quiet. As soon as we got home the phone was ringing. The voice on the other end told my dad that mom had passed away. My dad and step mom sat us down and told us. My brother and sister started crying. I did not. I think due to my young age I had no idea what that meant.

Shortly after while staying the weekend with my grandmother, a breast cancer survivor, I walked in on her changing and saw what looked like a huge hole on the left side of her chest. That image is forever stuck in my head. My mom was diagnosed with breast cancer at 34 and died at 37. My mom had a cousin that also died of breast cancer in her late thirties. In 2009 my grandmother had a recurrence of breast cancer. Sadly, she passed away at 78. My grandmother's sister also died in her seventies of breast cancer. Needless to say, since I was a teenager, I have felt that a breast cancer diagnosis was in my future.

Fast forward to October 2011. My older sister (41) goes to her gynecologist and he suggests that she take the BRCA test. She and I really knew nothing about it. She took the test and two weeks later went to her doctor's office for her results. He told her it was negative, folded the results up, placed them in an envelope and handed it to her.

Around that same time I saw a piece on Amy Shainman and BRCA testing on our local news. My husband also told me about a woman he worked with who was BRCA positive who had a prophylactic bilateral mastectomy (PBM), so it got me thinking. I made the appointment to meet with the genetic counselor, called my sister to tell her and that was that.

My sister gave me her test result to show the genetic counselor at my appointment. For whatever reason my sister never looked at her results after her doctor told her they were negative. When I went to meet with the genetic counselor she asked if anyone else in my family had been tested and if I had the results. I pulled out the envelope containing my sister's results and handed them to her. She looked at them and her mouth dropped open. She said. "I'm sorry to tell you this but your sister is not negative, she is positive." I looked at the paper and there in all caps and bold letters it said POSITIVE FOR

DELETRIOUS MUTATION. My first reaction was why did my sister not look at this? I started crying knowing my sister was thinking she was good to go and there was no chance that her children would have had this gene passed on to them and in reality she was positive. The genetic counselor saw my reaction and said we could postpone my test. I said, "No way," and took the test that day.

After taking the test I immediately went to my parent's house to let them know about my sister and we decided to drive to her house to tell her. She was devastated. We got her in to see the genetic counselor that day. She was already having some issues with her ovaries, which concerned me. She had a few cysts but nothing that her doctor was worried about. My sister met with a gynecological oncologist and decided to have an oophorectomy. She had her ovaries removed and the pathology came back that there was cancer. It was small and caught early. Up until this moment I was never a strong believer of the saying "everything happens for a reason" and I used to get annoyed when people would say it. Let's just say now I am a believer. Who knows what would have happened if she didn't give me her results? I am so thankful she found out when she did and her outcome is good.

About a week after taking the BRCA test, my results were in. I knew in my heart that it was positive and it was! That was November 7, 2011. After that I met with doctors to discuss my preventative options and went for a breast MRI. On December 23, 2011, I got the phone call that they saw something on the MRI and I would need a biopsy. This sent me into freak-out mode. I was not a fan of MRI and now I had to have another one with a biopsy. I had been getting mammograms since I was 24 and everything had always been fine. All I could think about was that this was going to be the time they came back and told me I had cancer. I had the biopsy and everything ended up being okay. I knew from the get-go that I would be having the PBM. The biopsy just reaffirmed it for me.

My husband and I have been together since 11th grade in high school and he has always known long before the BRCA test that if I ever had cancer, no matter how small I would have a mastectomy and hysterectomy. He understands and is so supportive. He has never questioned my decision and has been my cheerleader since day one. For me it hasn't been IF I get cancer it's been a matter of WHEN.

Losing my mother at such a young age has made me very fearful of not being here for my boys. I am grateful the BRCA test was available and I gained the knowledge to make these decisions. I look at the BRCA test and all of the prophylactic measures as a blessing. My nipple and skin sparing prophylactic bilateral mastectomy (PBM) was scheduled for May 16, 2012. I was excited to rid myself of the fear that has been living in me since I was a child. I was scared. I had never been in the hospital other than childbirth and never had general anesthesia. Those were my fears.

Fast forward to October 2012. I am about five months post-operative from my PBM. I am amazed at how well everything went. I woke up in the hospital not realizing I had already had the surgery. I thought they were getting ready to wheel me down, but in fact it was finished. I felt like a huge weight had been lifted from my shoulders. Recovery went smoothly and was much easier than I thought it would be. I didn't have very much pain at all, more of just a soreness/tightness. My drains came out at seven days and at three and a half weeks I told my doctor I was going back to work. Things are healing up nicely and my scars are already fading. I have my moments when I miss my real breasts but actually my new ones are more symmetrical than my real ones. In the end I did not do this for vanity. I did it to live and to see my boys grow up to become wonderful men like their father. I could be flat as a board and not care. The reconstruction is just a plus. I would have had the surgery even if reconstruction was not an option. I am however glad that it is an option because I think it helps with the recovery to feel more normal. I am planning to have my hysterectomy in the next two years. I am 33 years old and my husband and I are not planning on having anymore children but I just feel I should wait for now, as I am not looking forward to going into early menopause. I will definitely have my hysterectomy by the time I am 35.

My sister had several chemo treatments and had a complete hysterectomy a few weeks before my PBM. The pathology came back from her hysterectomy as cancer free. This goes back to the saying "everything happens for a reason". I am so thankful that her cancer was found early and that she was able to overcome it. She will be planning her PBM for the summer of 2013. It's amazing how quickly life changes. Last year I was in tears. This year my sister and I are both celebrating our lives as previvors, such an amazing feeling. I am thankful for the knowledge I have gained, amazed at how empowered I feel, and most of all, grateful that my sister is alive and cancer free.

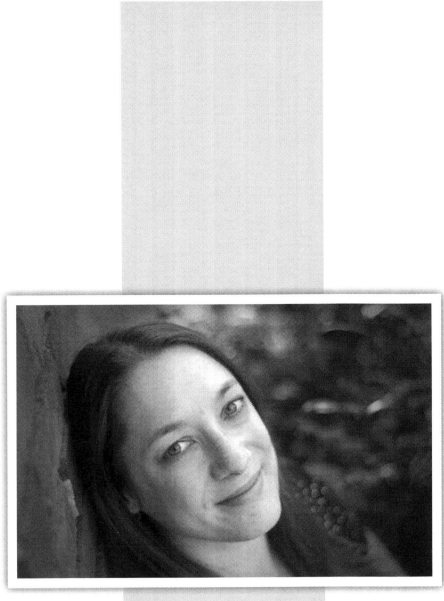

Sarah Kerstetter

BRCA1 Previvor, 31
Knoxville, Tennessee USA

Saving Myself

I guess my story began when I was eight years old. My mother and father sat my brother and I down at the kitchen table and delivered the news. After months of pain, discomfort, and being told her pain was plain old woman troubles, my mother was diagnosed with Stage IV ovarian cancer. Being eight I didn't truly understand what that meant, but I asked my mom if she was going to die. She said, "Not if I can help it." If you had known my mother you would know she didn't put up with anyone messing with her family.

I watched my mother bravely battle ovarian cancer off and on for the next eight years. My mother's personality was such that we didn't ask for help when we needed it because we took care of our own. I ended up giving up my childhood to cancer. At the age of eight, I became the "mother" of the household. Cooking, cleaning, and ironing were added to my daily schedule. Meanwhile, I saw the chemo ravage my mother's body and change the woman that I knew.

Throughout the fight my mother kept saying that she wanted to see her kids graduate. She was full of health when my brother, her first child, graduated high school and then watched him board a bus to leave for basic training as a member of the United States Air Force.

Two months later, at her yearly CAT scan she was told once again that the cancer had returned. I entered my sophomore year of high school and became my mother's caretaker. My dad was now the only one working and was gone the majority of the time. My brother was in the military, and my mom was dying. I had never in my life felt so alone.

Halfway through my sophomore year I came to Jesus out of fear, exhaustion, and pain. For once in my life I found peace and comfort in the world I was living in.

In December 1997 I came home from school to find my mother having difficulty breathing. I begged her to allow me to call the ambulance. She initially refused. She said she knew if she went in, she would never come home. After an hour of her struggling to breathe and me begging she relented. I watched the ambulance pull away from my home one more time. The last time.

My mother took her last breath on New Years Eve after telling me she loved me one last time. She was 48 years old.

I tell you this story, because without it, my story would never have begun.

I had always known I would have my ovaries removed when I was older. I had seen cancer rage through my mother's body and was determined to prevent it from happening to me. My fantastic Obstetrician was proactive with my health and suggested the BRCA test a time or two. I said no, because I felt I was already planning on taking the precautions so the genetic testing was unnecessary.

In 2008 I found myself pregnant. My first thought when the doctor announced we were having a boy was that he would not have to endure the worry of ovarian cancer. That same year I had the pleasure of teaching a young girl in my class whose mother was a genetic counselor. We got into a conversation one day about genetic testing and I again said I wasn't interested. However, a few months later while doing research on the health history of my family tree I discovered my grandmother had also died of ovarian cancer. I remember falling to the floor and begging Jesus to remove the fear that I suffered from so often. After crying and praying for some time, I realized what I needed to do.

I was tested in September of 2009 and knew the results before they were given to me. BRCA1 positive.

In the summer of 2011 I had a total hysterectomy. My doctor did an organ wash and tested everything that was removed. I can't tell you the relief that filled my soul when my doctor told me that everything came back free of cancer.

I have at this time, chosen surveillance for my breasts. I receive a breast MRI and a mammogram alternating every six months.

I have placed my trust in the hands of Christ and feel that my mother's journey helped me through my journey. I try to cherish every day that I get to spend with my husband and son. I know this story is long, but my mother isn't here to tell hers anymore, and her story is my story.

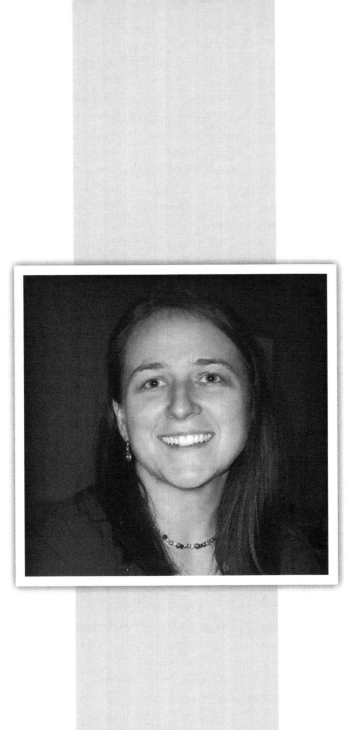

Emily Kelley

BRCA1 Previvor, 36
Foresthill, California USA

I Chose Prevention: My BRCA Story

I remember when I was 11 years old my aunt (dad's sister) was diagnosed with breast cancer at the age of 32. My cousins were seven and eight years old. I remember how weak she was, a shadow of who she used to be. It was like cancer sucked the life out of her. At 36, she died. I was 15 (my cousins were 11 and 12). That was when I started to worry that I could have breast cancer someday.

Meanwhile, when I was 14, my Grandma (mom's mom) was diagnosed with breast cancer at 63. She struggled for the next three years, until she was unable to live alone. The cancer had spread to her bones and liver. She moved in with us. It was so hard to see her deteriorate before our eyes, but I wouldn't trade those days for anything. How lucky we were (I have one younger sister and two younger brothers) to have our grandma at our house every day. Granted she was in a hospital bed in the living room most of the time, but someone was always there with her. She was in our house for almost a year before she died at the age of 67, after a four-year battle. This only added to my fear of getting breast cancer.

When I was 28, my mom was diagnosed with breast cancer at age 49. My world crashed. I remember how my aunt and grandma's battles ended and now it was happening to my mom. How could this be? She was the glue that held our family together. It was so hard on my dad, too. I remember when we were waiting for her to recover from her mastectomy so we could see her, he was crying. He said if they had to, they'd sell the house to cover the hospital bills and chemo costs. When I saw her after her surgery, she looked so weak and tired. It reminded me of my aunt and grandma. Even though I knew it was just the anesthesia, it was so hard to see my mom like that. She is always so strong. The next day, of course, she looked a lot more like herself. Good news: it's been eight years since her last chemo treatment (she had two rounds) and she's doing fabulous! She ended up having her other breast removed preventatively five years after her first.

When I was 28 I had my first yearly mammogram, as advised by my doctor. Every year I worried they would find something, but it was always clear, except for my super dense tissue. I also did monthly self-exams. My doctor recommended an annual MRI as well. I had my first one in July. He asked me every year since my mom's diagnosis if I would consider genetic testing, but I was never interested in knowing, mainly because I wouldn't do anything to prevent it. I really didn't want any surgeries. I had my kids, who were two and four years old when mom was diagnosed, so I was busy chasing toddlers around. So, this year when he asked me I said yes. Why not? There was a 50/50 chance it would be negative. So I met with a genetic counselor who explained how the BRCA test works, what the different results mean, and my options of surveillance versus preventative measures. Before I went to see her, I had to find out my family's cancer history. I found out that my Great Grandma on my mom's side also had breast cancer (diagnosed at 60, died at 73) and my Great Aunt on my dad's side also had breast cancer (diagnosed late 30's, died early 40's). So that gave me even more reason.

The day she called me with my results, I was at the local pool watching my kids swim with their friends. I was so shocked when she told me I am BRCA1 positive E1250X (3867G>T). It had been a couple weeks since I had seen her, so I had been researching like crazy. I felt like I was in school again. I am in a different stage in my life now than I was when my mom was diagnosed. I'm 36, my husband and I celebrated our 16th anniversary this summer and our boys are now 12 and 10 years old. It hit me that I'm the same age my aunt was when she died and my kids are about the same age my cousins were when they lost their mom. I want to be around to see them grow up. I want to be here with my husband.

Breast cancer has always been my #1, actually only, real cause for anxiety. I'm always worried about it. So I decided, the best choice for me would be the preventative route. It seems so extreme, but it will be worth it to reduce my risk to lower than an average woman's risk. Two weeks ago I had a bilateral salpingo oophorectomy and in two weeks I will have my prophylactic bilateral mastectomy with expanders to implants.

It was a struggle emotionally, at first, but now I'm doing a lot better. I still have my bad days. I just remind myself, that no matter how hard this is to go through, this is a gift. I watched my relatives get breast cancer, and most of those women didn't survive it. I can do something to prevent that from happening to my family and me. I am a previvor and proud to be one.

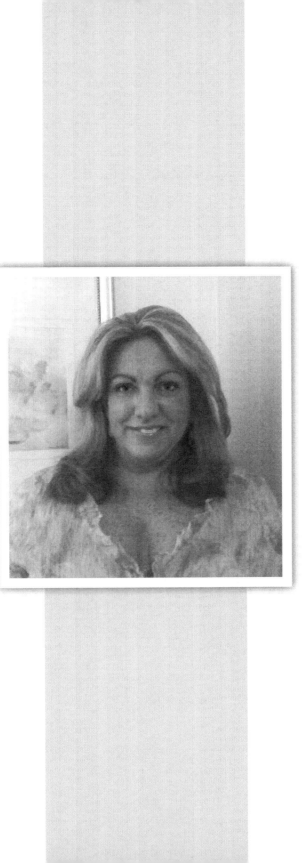

Lisa Marie Guzzardi

**Uninformative BRCA Negative Previvor
New York, USA**

My BRCA - less Story

I will remember when...

...I had my first encounter with breast cancer when my paternal grandma [aka Grammie] died at the age of 52. I was 10 years old and the "C" word was like the forbidden "F" word, never spoken. My maternal grandmother had died of breast cancer when I was five, but that's all I remember of her.

...My mom's sister developed breast cancer during my late teen-age years. She died a few years later. It was years following that when I learned my paternal great-grandmother died of ovarian cancer in her mid-forties, but I managed to conceal this and never thought much of it.

...I had my first surgical breast biopsy in 2005 to rule out Paget's Disease after unsuccessful treatment with a dermatologist. Thankfully, all was benign. This is when I first began to realize a hereditary/familial predisposition was a possibility.

...Exactly four months later, I found a lump in the same breast, but it too, was found to be benign.

...Several months passed and my younger cousin developed Stage II breast cancer at the age of 42.

...I tested negative for both BRCA mutations in March 2006, but nobody had yet tested for a possible mutation in my family.

...During the summer of 2006, just 15 months after my first biopsy, I finally told my breast surgeon I wanted to remove my breasts. I was facing another surgical excision on the opposite breast for new onset bloody nipple discharge. Again, I dodged the bullet with hyperplasia and papilloma findings.

...My maternal aunt was diagnosed with Stage IIIC ovarian cancer just before the Christmas holiday in 2007. She is also BRCA negative.

...I spent four and half years trying to make a decision for myself, but stuck with surveillance until my tolerance wore me down ever so tirelessly.

...I had an atypical mole removed on my left chest above the breast one month prior to my nipple-sparing mastectomy as per my surgical oncologist. All was okay. I also had an enlarged ovarian cyst that required repeat scans and blood work two months prior to my mastectomy date. I was on the verge of collapse, not knowing whether I would be having a prophylactic bilateral mastectomy (PBM) or a bilateral salpingo oophorectomy (BSO). Thankfully, I was given the green light to proceed with MY choice.

...On the morning of August 10, 2010, I was given a new life, a new beginning with a sense of renewal, hope and empowerment. I received a priceless gift that was denied to both maternal/paternal grandmothers, aunts and cousins. Each one of these family members suffered from hereditary breast cancer. I refused to become another potential victim of this devastating familial disease.

As a result, I had a risk reducing bilateral total skin nipple/areola sparing bilateral mastectomy followed by immediate breast reconstruction. Not only does this "cutting edge" procedure allow many women a dramatic risk reduction, but it also provides us with a huge sense of normalcy and amazing outcomes, without compromising oncological safety. This is also in accordance with the latest research findings that continually demonstrate a broader acceptance and approval within the oncology community. It was the expertise, amazing skill, compassion and trust with my breast surgical oncologist, Richard Shapiro, that made this possible for myself. My plastic surgeon, Nolan Karp, was equally impressive by fully restoring my breasts with such skillful artistry, leaving me with a natural appearance. Together, they have formed a unique and highly skilled partnership. Many women, whose lives have been touched by breast cancer, whether they are a "previvor" like myself or survivors, have this gentler option. I truly feel as though I have lost nothing, but my risks.

...Another cousin was diagnosed with advanced breast cancer at the age of 53 just one month after my PBM. She continues to battle the disease without an identifiable BRCA mutation.

...Sadly, my aunt died of ovarian cancer after a courageous four and a half year battle in June 2011.

...I had a risk reducing BSO performed in October 2011 after waiting a year following my PBM and after three years of close surveillance under the brilliant guidance and direction of Elizabeth Poynor, GYN Oncologist.

...In March of 2012, I landed on the Pink Moon, after Nicki Boscia Durlester found me somewhere over the rainbow. My home sweet home filled with the loveliest lovelies whom share an endless passion for each other, like no other place. I am forever blessed by Nicki and for the empowering venue she created for all high-risk women. She is the biggest piece of heaven here on earth.

...August 10, 2012 arrives, my second anniversary and many many more yet to come, my new birthday. I feel fortunate and ever so blessed for an amazing journey. For those who are also previvors, may we all previve together, forever more. And for those less fortunate, may you always be a survivor, true inspirations for all of us. Finally, for all of our loved ones who have died of hereditary cancers or any cancer, together we will always remember you. We shall never forget how much our lives were touched by your brief and powerful presence as we seek a cure to end the deadly curse once and for all. ♥

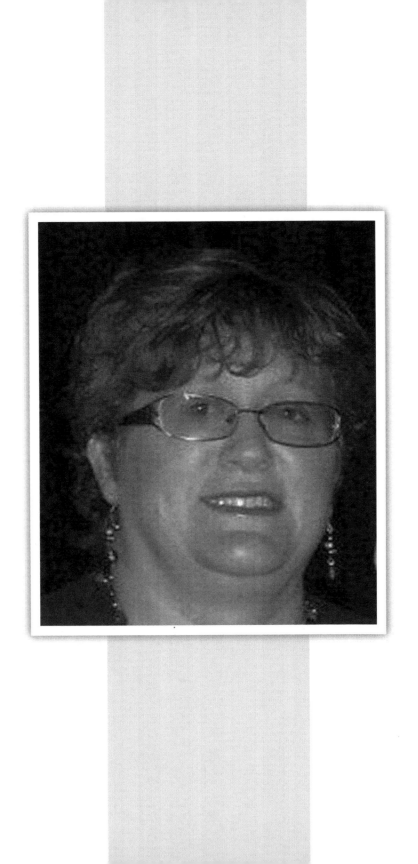

Kristi Ward McMurtry

BRCA (True) Negative, 44
McLeansboro, Illinois USA

BRCA1 and My Family

My maternal grandma married young, at age 13. By the time she was 20 she had been married twice and had children with both husbands. Over the next several years she added to her family giving birth to a total of fourteen children, raising thirteen to adulthood.

In 1987 one of her younger daughters, my aunt, was diagnosed with Stage I breast cancer. She had one breast and thirty-two lymph nodes removed. Seven of the lymph nodes were positive for cancer. She had reconstruction followed by chemo and has been cancer free for 25 years. In 2011, she had prophylactic surgeries including a mastectomy of her other breast and a bilateral oophorectomy.

In 2000 at the age of 70, Grandma was diagnosed with Stage IIIC ovarian cancer. The doctors removed an eight-pound tumor. They said it was not a familial cancer because of Grandma's age at diagnosis. Grandma fought a long, hard battle for almost eight years. She often said the cancer would not kill her and planned to live until

96. Unfortunately Grandma passed away on September 10, 2008 at the age of 78.

Last year, 24 years after her initial diagnosis of Stage1 breast cancer, my aunt tested positive for the BRCA1 gene mutation. That one piece of information sent our family on quite a journey. Shortly thereafter I found out one of my cousins, who is battling inflammatory breast cancer, also tested positive. She is the daughter of my mom's brother. Since her mother passed away from ovarian cancer it was initially unknown as to which side of the family carried the BRCA1 mutation. One would have thought that it was her mother who passed down the mutation, when in fact it was her father.

I tested for the BRCA1 gene in June 2011. I received my results a few weeks later on my 43rd birthday. The nurse at my doctor's office said she did not understand the report, but she would read the results to me. I knew exactly what it meant. I had tested positive for the BRCA1 mutation. I told my husband and began to cry. I called my mom. While I was on the phone with my mother call waiting clicked in. It was the nurse at my doctor's office calling back to tell me she had read the wrong report. She did not know where my report was. I waited for what seemed like an eternity. What a great birthday present! Just as I was about to call the doctor's office back, the phone rang. They had found my report and I was negative for the BRCA1 mutation. I don't know how many times I asked, "Are you sure?" What a roller coaster ride! I was emotionally worn out.

Two weeks later I met with my doctor. I was still in doubt and wondering if I had been given the correct report. Even after receiving it in writing, I still wonder if it's really true. I had decided if I had the BRCA1 mutation I would have the prophylactic bilateral mastectomy and reconstruction. Now what do I do? I should be thankful and I am, but I struggle with the guilt that I am negative when so many members of my family are positive. Why am I negative? These are the questions no one can answer. It's the difference between a flip of a coin. Just dumb luck. Each family member has a 50/50 chance of having the genetic mutation. I won the coin toss.

To date four of my first cousins tested for the BRCA1 mutation. Two are negative and two are positive for the BRCA1 mutation. My mom and five of her sisters have also tested. All of them are carriers of the BRCA1 gene mutation. The remaining brothers who are alive have not tested. Three of my aunts had prophylactic surgeries, two of them without complications. Another aunt will be starting her surgery journey in the next few weeks.

We now know that Grandma passed down the gene in our family. It may seem extreme or unfair to some that my family has so many members dealing with this. Many of us believe it is a blessing the Lord has given us. It is an opportunity for my family members to make a choice to have prophylactic surgeries to greatly reduce their risk of breast and ovarian cancer. I take comfort in knowing this journey has brought our family closer together.

I know the Lord is with us no matter what. I know with His help, we can do all things. And we know that all things work together for good for those who love God, to those who are the called according to His purpose. Romans 8:28 NKJV

Bad things may befall us, but if we allow and seek His will, the Lord will help us through. Sometimes we get so caught up wallowing in our pit of misery we forget to look and see what we can learn and what we can use to help others in similar situations.

In Memoriam

There are stars
whose radiance is visible on earth
though they have long been extinct.

There are people
whose brilliance continues to light the world
though they are no longer among the living.

These lights are particularly bright when the night is dark.
They light the way for humanity.

~Hannah Senesh~

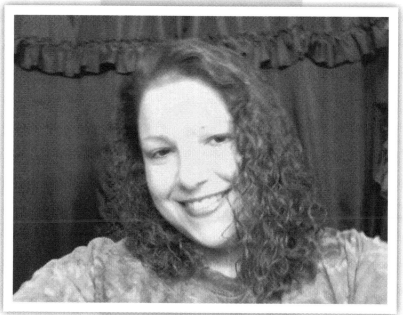

Linda Ritzco Cieszkowski

January 13, 1974 – July 18, 2012

May Smith

December 2, 1980 – July 22, 2012

May's Story

BRCA1 and 2, Triple Negative Breast Cancer
Capetown, SOUTH AFRICA

Where to start this is the question? Suppose at the beginning but that will take forever. So I will start only 32 years ago, LOL, seeing that I am 32 years old.

I didn't really know my grandma on my father's side. She died when I was still very young due to ovarian cancer. Grandma on mom's side is still alive as well as is grandpa. But grandma's family is full of cancer. Somehow she managed not to get any, thank heavens!

I first felt a lump in my left breast at the age of 29, but didn't pay much attention to it. Went for mammogram that said I had very dense breast tissue. Ultrasound however showed a tumor. But after a fine needle biopsy they said it is nothing. Doctor spoke about BRCA testing and I said fine. Came back positive for both BRCA1 and 2. Doctor explained how rare this was and spoke about preventive operations.

I said there is NO way and that I would go for screening every six months. During that time my dad passed away after a massive heart attack. The lump in my left breast got bigger and bigger and made me scared and I skipped my next screening. Also suffered from depression after my dad and even spent three weeks in the hospital.

So about a year after the first mammogram I went back and got diagnosed with Breast Cancer Stage III. Tumor was big and we did chemo to shrink it. After 12 rounds of chemo I was given a month break before my double mastectomy. It was the worst time of my life. After chemo I just couldn't believe that I had to lose my boobs as well!! I loved my boobs! Kept on thinking that I will wake up and it was all just a bad dream. How could this happen to me I am way to young?

Driving to hospital the morning of my operation I kept on listening to a Hillsong song, called Healer. Knowing that God will heal me and take away this pain. After that came radiation which wasn't so bad for me.

Now I am 32 years old! Just got news that big C is back in lymph nodes. (was clean for 1 year, 2 months and 6 days) I am between a rock and a hard place at the moment. Went to see a homeopathic doctor earlier and I am thinking about going the homeopathic route. I don't think I can do chemo again. My family is in the middle of a huge crisis and adding this news is not going to work. Going an alternative route I can do this on my own. I trust that God will help me get through this again, otherwise He wouldn't send this my way once again.

I still have hysterectomy or oophorectomy ahead of me but first need to cross this cancer bridge.

So my journey is not over but I know this is making all of us the strongest most amazing ladies ever!

May's Final Message
to the Pink Moon Lovelies

Written on July 22, 2012, the day she passed away.

Dearest Pink Moon Lovelies,

I joined this very special group about a year ago. Was something like 250 members. And boy did we grow. Each new Lovely had a place in my heart. And as I come to the end of my journey I want all of you to know the following:

• No one ever said life was going to be easy, we on this group or rather family know that.

• Always support the other Lovelies, even if in your heart you're thinking, just get over it. Their problems are just as big as yours, and where-as you don't want to share, the Lovely complaining about something "small" had the guts to do it.

This group was created by the most amazing, loving, kind, wonderful person I've ever met. We have formed a relationship that few people understand. We have become like mother and daughter in more ways than one. I mean, I even spoke to my mama about sex!

This group brings people from all over the world together, all religions, all political parties, and all races. So here we need to tolerate each other and their opinions. Believe me in the end it doesn't matter...

I have been going through so many emotions lately and thought to myself after I spoke to my mama last night that it's all okay in the end, if it's not okay it's not the end. Meaning this is not the end, I'll get a chance to meet all of you one day. So am I okay with dying, NO! But I'm not dying; I'm going to start living. And I didn't give up, cause I don't know how to. I'm winning all the way. If this is becoming confusing, try talking sense while being on so much pain meds.

I have kept a scrapbook of my Pink Moon Family. Every uplifting post is in there. A short description of those of you who wrote your story down. I ended round about when we reached 803. Started feeling too tired then. I also kept a daily prayer list and I had my mama and Melbert on the top of that list everyday. I hope some of you will start making a daily prayer list, I know some already do. I believe that by doing that we have the power to change things. You Lovelies are my family and I know when I go to sleep later I'll have all of you in the room next to me, guiding me towards the mountain top, where the most beautiful view will await me....

Nuff said!

Eulogy for May

By NICKI BOSCIA DURLESTER

The sun has set in South Africa and our angel, May Smith, has been laid to rest. Three eulogies were read at her service today, which took place in a vineyard surrounded by mountains. There were several hundred people in attendance. May's dear friend, Christelle, wrote, "I have never seen so much love in one place like today."

These were my parting words to my South African daughter

When Jerry Cowley wrote and said May wanted me to write something for her funeral my initial reaction was... how can I do my angel justice? May Smith was the most selfless person I have ever known. She added depth and meaning to my life with passion, courage, strength and grace that is beyond words. My only regret is that we met in the final chapter of hers. Time is the real bling-bling of life and I wanted more with May. We met over the Internet just a year ago when May joined a Facebook Group I moderate. May quickly became an active member. I instantly gravitated towards her unique voice filled with endless love for living and compassion for others.

I can't recall when we began calling each other mama and daughter, but I do remember from the beginning that is how I felt about her…. a daughter I met later in life that was always meant to be mine. We shared over 800 private Facebook messages and emails including photographs from recent days of May and her beloved cats, Tease and Sassy. She wrote so lovingly of her dear friend, Christelle, who has been by her side since they met during chemo and remained there every step of this arduous journey. She worried so much about Christelle. In the end she made sure Christelle was not alone when she called her "crazy" (May's word not mine) and beloved Aunt Diane in her final days to be there for her sweet friend. May wrote, "My aunt is funny and all dramatic. Walked into the room and asked me if I'm still alive, said I looked dead already! WTF? Then she started crying and I started laughing, so all good. It's good to have her here, told her I'll let her know when to come. And she is very grateful." I am grateful too, Diane, that you added levity and love when May needed it most.

I want to take this moment to personally thank Christelle for everything she did for May. I have never known a more devoted, caring friend who slept by May's side in the hospital and in recent days in a chair in her room. May loved the fact that she could always count on her. And oh how she loved her Jerry, who it turns out loved her too, confessing this secret at the Mad Hatter dinner party. That meant the world to May. In a different place and time I do believe she would have walked down the aisle with him. He shared her love of surfing and made her the best space cakes in town. May spoke so lovingly of Karien, her sweet, sensitive friend who brought so much joy to her life, so grateful she was there in the end. She wrote to me about her going away party from work and sent me the speech she read to all of her co-workers. She had a special fondness in her heart for Pierre, the owner of the company she took so much pride in, who had been so good to her when she was ill. She couldn't believe she was retiring before him when he was double her age. She had learned so much from Pierre and he in turn had learned about compassion from her. She said her co-workers were more like a family than a business and she would always treasure the fact that they shaved their heads in solidarity for her when she lost hers during chemo. She loved her work and had someday dreamed of owning her own company. I have no doubt that she would have.

In recent days I asked May what were the happiest moments in her life. This is what she wrote...

Happy moments: Getting my own surfboard!

The day my mom came home from hospital with my sister. Amazing to see a baby and I played with her like she was a doll, my mom had to step in a number of times or my sis might not have been here.

Flying all over S.A. to take part in athletics. One very special trip with my high school musical group, got my first kiss during that trip, 15years old!

Family vacations every year during July to Natal, it's winter then, but still warm there. I have a sensitive skin, so we couldn't go during summer.

Getting a scholarship to varsity, my 4 years there! Amazing friends, amazing times!!! Going on endless road trips in search of the perfect wave.

Buying my own house.

The last Christmas my dad was still alive. Spent it as a family at the beach.

Seeing snow for the first time in my life at age 22, wow, it still amazes me! So pure and clean.

Late night or early morning surfing sessions with Jer and the gang. Them always being worried if I tried something crazy. And then kicking their asses at it!

Bungy jumping at Bloukrans, it's fantastic!! Scared shitless, but so glad I did it and that the rope didn't snap, lol.

Shark cage diving the weekend before I got diagnosed first, can't describe that feeling!!

My last chemo and having met so many new friends. Did I say my last chemo already??!!??

Meeting my mama, years to late but actually at the perfect stage.

And then weird as it may sound, I'm happy now. I get a chance that only a few people get. Time to reflect, time to plan, time to prepare.

In one of her final messages written after we spoke on the phone the day before she died, May wrote...I have been going through so many emotions lately and thought to myself after I spoke to my mama last night that it's all okay in the end, if it's not okay, it's not the end. Meaning this is not the end. I'll get a chance to meet all of you one day. So am I okay with dying? NO! But I'm not dying, I'm going to start living. And I didn't give up, cause I don't know how to. I'm winning all the way!!

And that's my girl... she reached the mountaintop and saw the most spectacular view and took her leap of faith. I am so proud of you, May. So proud of the way you lived your life. I am hugely blessed to have shared this journey with you. I didn't let go my love, I'm still holding on. Until we meet again I will look for the signs and I promise I will smell all of the roses along the way. Your American mama will love you madly with all of my heart forever and beyond.

ACKNOWLEDGMENTS

NICKI BOSCIA DURLESTER

I love the Pink Moon Lovelies! I am grateful to each and every one of them for their encouragement, inspiration, humor and love. They fill my soul.

Thank you for telling your stories. Women can feel lost in this process whether they have just been diagnosed with breast or ovarian cancer or they are considering prophylactic surgery. Your journeys will let them know they are not alone and will highlight the fact that every person's experience is unique. Each woman's choice is her own to make. Keeping telling your stories. You will save lives! And remember to drink your Matcha!!

A special thank you to the team of contributors on this book.

Melissa Johnson Voight, thank you for saying yes. You are the perfect partner on Pink Moon. You lift our spirits every day with your inspirational posts and kind and encouraging words. I know I can always count on you. Thank you for editing the photographs for this book and for allowing me to bounce ideas off you, sometimes the same ones over and over again. You have the patience of a saint. I may have hung the moon, but you painted it pink. Love you, Melbert, to the moon and back!

Susan Long Martucci, I loved every minute of the endless hours we spent editing this book. We laughed, cried, and fretted about each word. I just hope and pray there are no typos in this book. Thank you for reaching out and finding me. You are my confidante and treasured friend. I know Rose and Bianchina are smiling down on us! Love you Martucci! Survivors 'r us!

Maria Flodin, in the midst of your own recovery you volunteered to help with this book. It still amazes me how well you write in English, considering Swedish is your first language. Thank you for your work on the Glossary of Terms. More importantly thank you for being my Swedish angel. You will always be the other half of M&M, Inc. My love to you!

Lisa Marie Guzzardi, thank you for being our resident nurse on Pink Moon. The Lovelies rely on you for your expert advice and compassionate spirit. You have made a huge impact on Pink Moon and will forever be known as the soul twin of our beloved Zelda Nagel. Many thanks for researching and compiling the Glossary of Terms and Links. You will always be the Curly to my Moe. Nothin' but Stooge love for you!

Shera Delia, from the first time I saw your painting, *Spring Forward*, I knew it had to be the cover of our book. It drew me in and inspired me to complete this project. You are a gifted artist. You took your own diagnosis, treatment and recovery and allowed it to inspire you to new heights. Thank you for designing the cover of The Pink Moon Lovelies, Empowering Stories of Survival. I love it!

Michael Pauldine, thank you for your profound and powerful quote at the beginning of this book. You are one of a few men brave enough to call yourself a Lovely. Your recommendations on Pink Moon about healthy lifestyle choices are deeply appreciated. Prevention is key on this war on cancer. Many thanks for motivating us with your pearls of wisdom. I will never forget what you did for me during my recovery. You healed me!

My deepest gratitude to my breast surgeon, Dr. Kristi Funk. When I asked Dr. Funk if she would contribute to this book, she immediately said yes. No hesitation! Speaks volumes about the kind of woman she is. Dr. Funk, it's no secret you are a rock star breast surgeon, but you are also an extraordinary human being. Thank you for the important work you do. Let's Save Lives is the motto of Pink Lotus Breast Center. Thank you for saving mine! Forever grateful my friend!

My heartfelt appreciation and respect to my plastic surgeon, Dr. Jay Orringer, who put me back together again. Dr. Orringer is a gifted physician and a mensch of a man, who still makes house calls. His attentive and comforting bedside manner combined with his skillful artistry as a plastic surgeon are unparalleled. Thank you Dr. O! I will always remember your kindness.

A special acknowledgment to Dr. James Waisman, my brilliant, kind and compassionate oncologist. Thank you Dr. Waisman for fielding all of my questions for the Pink Moon Lovelies. Your immediate follow-up and thoughtful responses mean the world to me. It cannot be easy having a patient whose thirst for knowledge and continued questioning never ends. Many thanks for your patience and understanding. I'm coming with you to City of Hope!

And now to the three most important people in my life.... my husband, Alan, and children Ally and Matthew.

Big Al, thank you for your support while I toiled over this book. I know it hasn't been easy, but as always you cheered me on every step of the way. I'm sure you never expected me to turn my diagnosis into my life's work. But, you also know that once I get a hold of something I never let it go. I gotcha then, I gotcha now. I love you Alan!

Ally Bianchina, grazie bella for being a wonderful daughter and best friend. You light up my life more than you'll ever know. Thank you for writing your heartfelt story. I know it took great courage and I hope it was cathartic. I am confident you will make decisions that are right for you and you will move on with the rest of your life. This time and place will not define you. It will enrich you. You are a happy person. Smile always my love. *T' iamo!*

Matthew Hunter, I know every time you turned around I was sitting at the computer immersed in this project. Thank you for your patience and for all those nights I ordered in for you and Dad. No time to cook as I worked on this book. Mama will be back in the kitchen soon. I love you boychick! There is no one I would rather sneak into the garage with and eat See's Candies. Our secret!

When I wrote <u>Beyond the Pink Moon</u> I thought a few close friends and family might read it. I never dreamed my book would travel around the globe and lead to this compelling collection of stories from Lovelies around the world. Anything is possible if you believe. Beyond the Pink Moon I found The Pink Moon Lovelies.

MELISSA JOHNSON VOIGHT

I would like to take this opportunity to thank the Pink Moon Lovelies for your encouragement and daily support. It has been a joy each day to see how you reach out to the members in Beyond the Pink Moon, with open arms and compassion. You came into my life in God's perfect timing. I always prayed that I would be able to use my journey to help others and I was led to you. Thus began not only friendships, but a sense of belonging and family. Thank you for your acceptance, love and support.

To Nicki Boscia Durlester, my dear sweet friend. Thank you for reaching out to me and allowing me this wonderful opportunity to be your partner on the Pink Moon. You are greatly loved and admired. You are someone I can always turn to for advice, support and understanding. Our meeting was no accident, but a godsend. Your own personal journey evolved into a place of beauty and opened the door for many to call their home. May you have every happiness today, tomorrow and always.

I would like to thank the loved ones in my life that have helped me along the way in my personal journey. First of all, thank you to my husband and best friend, Bert Voight. Your love and support during these past two years has meant so much to me. Thank you for embracing the "new normal" and accepting me and loving me through it all. Thank you for honoring our vows that we made before God, " for better or worse, in sickness and in health." I love you!

Secondly, I would like to extend my love and deep appreciation to my children, Devan and Kelsey. I know this wasn't easy for the both of you to completely understand every detail of this proactive choice, but you understood enough that I was doing this to be here for you and our family. Thank you for making every effort to help me and love me through it all.

Thank you to my cousin, Karen, for lovingly testing for the BRCA gene, when you were diagnosed with breast cancer and fighting your own battle. God used you to save my life and the lives of our family members. You were my hero! I will love you always and I carry this torch, proudly, in your memory. Until heaven!

To my sister, Kim. Thank you for being there for me from day one, when we received the news of the BRCA results, until my very last appointment. You always insisted on being right there with me, every step of the way. For that, I am forever grateful. Thank you for being strong for me, and encouraging me to move forward. I admire you greatly and I love you dearly!

To my parents for sacrificing their own needs to be with me. Mom, for staying with me for weeks on end, as I recovered from surgery. I am certain it wasn't easy, but you never once complained. You are a vision of grace and showed God's love in all that you did. I hope you both know how much I appreciate you and love you!

To my in-laws for attending every surgery, no matter how early it was. It always gave me a sense of comfort to know that you were there when I went in for surgery and when I woke up. Thank you for never questioning me, but trusting me that I was doing what God had called me to do. I love you!

I would like to thank my surgeons and their assistants. Thank you for making it easy to trust you and your abilities to extend my life. Thank you for always being open and honest with me, and looking out for my best interests. I thank God for the abilities, the knowledge and the blessings that He has bestowed upon each one of you.

Thank you Lord for bringing me safely on the other side of this journey, as you promised. Though it was not always easy or as I had planned, your purpose was fulfilled, and for that I am grateful. Thank you for making beauty from the ashes. Thank you for the friends that you brought into my life along the way. I could have never imagined my life being this wonderful. Thank you for your faithfulness and for always keeping your promises.

GLOSSARY of TERMS

ADH

Atypical ductal hyperplasia (ADH) is a proliferative change in which the cells that line the milk ducts of the breasts experience abnormal growth. It is a marker for women who may have a risk factor for developing breast cancer in the future.

ALH

An abnormal appearing growth of cells within lobules of the breast that is associated with an increased risk of subsequent breast cancer.

BC

Breast cancer

Bilateral

On both sides of the body. For instance, 'Bilateral Mastectomies' means the removal of both breasts

BM, BPM

Bilateral Mastectomies or Bilateral Prophylactic (or preventive) Mastectomies

BRCA1

A gene on chromosome 17 that normally helps to suppress cell growth. A person who inherits certain mutations (changes) in a BRCA1 gene has a higher risk of getting breast, ovarian, prostate, and other types of cancer

BRCA2

A gene on chromosome 13 that normally helps to suppress cell growth. A person who inherits certain mutations (changes) in a BRCA2 gene has a higher risk of getting breast, ovarian, prostate, pancreatic and other types of cancer.

BRCA Positive

A positive test result generally indicates that a person has inherited a known harmful mutation in BRCA1 or BRCA2 and, therefore, has an increased risk of developing certain cancers. However, a positive test result provides information only about a person's risk of developing cancer. It cannot determine whether an individual will actually develop cancer or when. Not all women who inherit a harmful BRCA1 or BRCA2 mutation will develop breast or ovarian cancer.

BRCA (True) Negative

Interpretation depends on whether or not someone in the tested person's family is known to carry a harmful *BRCA1* or *BRCA2* mutation. If someone in the family has a known mutation, testing other family members for the same mutation can provide information about their cancer risk. If a person tests negative for a known family mutation, it is unlikely that they have an inherited susceptibility to cancer associated with *BRCA1* or *BRCA2*. Such a test result is called a "true negative."

BRCA Uninformative Negative

In cases in which a family has a history of breast and/or ovarian cancer and no known mutation in BRCA1 or BRCA2 has been previously identified, a negative test result is then termed "uninformative". It is not possible to tell whether an individual has a harmful BRCA1 or BRCA2 mutation that was not detected by testing (a "false negative") or whether the result is a true negative. In addition, it is also possible for some families to have a yet unidentified mutation in a gene other than BRCA1 or BRCA2 that increases their cancer risk but is not detectable by the test(s) used.

Breast Density

Breast density is a measure used to describe the proportion of the different tissues that make up a woman's breasts. Breast density compares the area of breast and connective tissue seen on a mammogram to the area of fat.

BSE

Breast self-examination

BSO

Bilateral salpingo-oophorectomy (removal of both tubes and both ovaries)

CA-125

A blood test used to detect signs of ovarian cancer, monitors the response to OVCA treatment.

CBE

Clinical breast examination; a breast exam performed by a health-care professional

Contralateral

Having to do with the opposite side of the body

DCIS

Ductal carcinoma in situ, a non-invasive type of breast cancer found in the lining of a breast duct.

DIEP

Diep Inferior Epigastric Perforator, a type of breast flap reconstruction surgery

DPM

Double prophylactic mastectomies); same as BPM, PBM or risk re-ducing mastectomies

Dual-energy X-ray absorptionmetry (DXA scan)

Best technique to measure bone density. Typically used to diagnose and follow osteoporosis.

ERT

Estrogen replacement therapy

Fibroadenoma

A benign (non-cancerous) breast tumor that is made of glandular and fibrous breast tissue. Very common in pre-menopausal women, and they can occur in groups.

Flap

A type of breast reconstruction using the body's own tissue

FNA

Fine needle aspirate (a technique for sampling breast tissue by placing a needle into the breast and removing cells).

GYN/ONC

A pelvic oncologist surgeon who specializes in treating cancers of the female reproductive organs and also treats women with predisposing risk factors.

Herceptin

A drug used to treat breast cancer that is HER2-positive (expresses the human epidermal growth factor receptor 2).

HER2: HER2/neu (human epidermal growth factor receptor 2), also called ErbB2

A protein that appears on the surface of some breast cancer cells. This protein is an important part of the pathway for cell growth and survival.

HER2 Positive

Describes cancer cells that have too much of a protein called HER2 on their surface.

HRT

Hormone replacement therapy

Hyst

Hysterectomy, or removal of the uterus

IBC

Inflammatory Breast Cancer

IDC

Invasive Ductal Carcinoma

Intraductal Breast Papilloma

A benign (not cancer), wart-like growth in a milk duct of the breast. It is usually found close to the nipple and may cause a discharge from the nipple.

IVF

In Vitro Fertilization: a fertility treatment where the women's eggs are removed and fertilized in a test tube.

LAVH

Laparoscopic-assisted vaginal hysterectomy

LCIS

Lobular cancer in situ, a noninvasive change in the lobules of the breast that increases the risk of developing breast cancer in both breasts.

Lymphedema

A condition of localized fluid retention and tissue swelling caused by a compromised lymphatic system that generally occurs in one of your arms. It can happen in both. Lymphedema is most commonly caused by the removal of or damage to your lymph nodes as a part of cancer treatment and surgery.

Mammaprint

Developed by Agendia in the Netherlands, a test that is used to help predict whether breast cancer will recur. The test looks at the activity of 70 different genes in a fresh tissue sample of breast cancer in women who have early-stage breast cancer that has not spread to the lymph nodes.

Mammo

Mammogram

MRI

Magnetic Resonance Imaging: a technique for looking for abnormalities such as cancer using magnetic fields. Breast MRI is typically recommended as a screening tool for breast cancer in high-risk women and is often used to follow up on a breast abnormality seen on mammogram.

Mutation Carrier

A person who has a mutated (changed) copy of a (BRCA) gene. This change may cause a disease in that person or in his or her children.

NCI

National Cancer Institute

NIH

National Institute of Health

NSM

Nipple/areola sparing mastectomy

Omentum

A fold of peritoneum connecting the stomach with the other abdominal organs.

Oncotype DX

Developed by Genomic Health in the United States, is a twenty-one-gene assay done on a frozen tissue sample that provides an individualized prediction of chemotherapy benefit and ten-year distant recurrence in certain women with early stage breast cancer.

Ooph

Oophorectomy, or surgical removal of the ovaries

OVCA

Ovarian cancer

Paget's Disease

A rare type of breast cancer involving the skin of the nipple and usually the areola.

PBM

Surgery to lower the risk of developing breast cancer by removing one or both breasts before disease develops. Also called preventive or risk reducing mastectomy.

PET Scan

A procedure in which a small amount of radioactive glucose (sugar) is injected into a vein, and a scanner is used to make detailed, computerized pictures that can be used to find cancer cells in the body.

PICC Line

A thin, flexible tube that is inserted into a vein in the upper arm and guided (threaded) into a large vein near the heart. Used to give intravenous fluids, blood transfusions, and chemotherapy and other drugs, and for taking blood samples.

Previvor

Individual who is a survivor of a predisposition to cancer but who hasn't had the disease. This group includes people who carry a hereditary mutation, a family history of cancer, or some other predisposing factor.

Port-A-Cath

An implanted device through which blood may be withdrawn and drugs may be infused without repeated needle sticks.

PS

Abbreviation for 'plastic surgeon'

PSO
Prophylactic salpingo-oophorectomy (removal of tubes and ovaries)

Recon
Reconstruction, or breast reconstructive surgery

Revision
A type of surgical procedure, which may be done as a follow-up to a prior operation, such breast reconstruction.

Salpingectomy
Surgical removal of fallopian tubes

SSM
Skin sparing mastectomy

TAH
Total abdominal hysterectomy

Sono
Sonogram (ultrasound)

TAH
Total abdominal hysterectomy

TNBC
Triple Negative Breast Cancer, also called ER-negative PR-negative HER2/neu-negative breast cancer

TRAM

Transverse rectus abdominous myocutaneous flap: a type of reconstructive surgery where fat and muscle from the abdomen are used to recreate breast tissue.

TVH

Total vaginal hysterectomy

TVU

Transvaginal ultrasound

Unilateral

Refers to single sided, as a single mastectomy

U/S

Ultrasound; or ultrasonographic examination

LINKS

The Facebook group Beyond The Pink Moon
https://www.facebook.com/groups/BeyondthePinkMoon/

Beyond the Pink Moon, A Memoir of Legacy, Loss and Survival
http://beyondthepinkmoon.com/

American Society of Plastic Surgeons
http://www.plasticsurgery.org/Reconstructive-Procedures/Breast-Reconstruction.html

Basser Research Center for BRCA
https://www.penncancer.org/basser/

Bright Pink
http://www.brightpink.org/

BRCA Sisterhood
https://www.facebook.com/groups/brcasisterhood/?fref=ts

The Breast Reconstruction Guidebook, 3rd Edition
http://www.breastrecon.com/index.html

Center for Restorative Breast Surgery, New Orleans
http://www.breastcenter.com/

FORCE: Facing Our Risk of Cancer Empowered
http://www.facingourrisk.org/

Fox Chase Cancer Center
http://www.fccc.edu/

Kristi Funk, MD, FACS, Surgical Breast Oncologist
Founder and Director, Pink Lotus Breast Center
http://www.pinklotusbreastcenter.com/

Joan Karvell Cancer Center at Pennsylvania Hospital
http://www.pennmedicine.org/pahosp/cancer/

Nolan Karp, MD, Plastic Surgeon
http://www.kcnyplasticsurgery.com/

MammaPrint
http://www.agendia.com

North American Menopause Society
http://www.menopause.org/home

National Cancer Institute, Breast Cancer:
Prevention, Genetics, Causes
http://www.cancer.gov/cancertopics/prevention-genetics-causes/breast

Oncotype DX
http://www.oncotypeDX.com

Jay Orringer, MD, Plastic Surgeon
http://www.drorringer.com/

Elizabeth Poyner, MD/PhD GYN Oncologist
www.drelizabethpoynor.com

Previvors and Survivors
http://previvorsandsurvivors.com

Richard L. Shapiro, MD, Surgical Breast Oncologist
http://www.med.nyu.edu/biosketch/shapir01

Made in the USA
Lexington, KY
23 March 2013